Dr Alice Boyes is an emotions expert and a popular blogger for *Psychology Today*. Her research has been published by The American Psychological Association.

D1394329

Praise for

THE ANXIETY TOOLKIT

"*The Anxiety Toolkit* provides quick, simple and practical tips that the anxious person can use now."
—Robert L. Leahy, PhD, director of the American Institute for Cognitive Therapy

"In this innovative handbook, Dr. Boyes identifies common habits that underlie different types of anxiety. She then offers clear strategies to drop the fight and become more gentle with ourselves. If anxiety has limited your life in any way, this book is an excellent place to start the healing process."
—Christopher Germer, PhD, clinical instructor at Harvard Medical School, coeditor of *Mindfulness and Psychotherapy*, and author of *The Mindful Path to Self-Compassion*

"*The Anxiety Toolkit* is an investment in wellness. Based on years of clinical practice and research, Dr. Alice Boyes has written a real-world roadmap for all of us who struggle with making decisions and feeling stuck."
—Chris Guillebeau, *New York Times* bestselling author of *The Happiness of Pursuit* and *The $100 Startup*

THE
ANXIETY
TOOLKIT

Strategies for managing your anxiety
so you can get on with your life

DR ALICE BOYES

piatkus

PIATKUS

First published in the US in 2015 as a PERIGEE book by Penguin Group (USA) LLC
First published in Great Britain in 2015 by Piatkus

3 5 7 9 10 8 6 4

Copyright © 2015 by Alice Boyes

The moral right of the author has been asserted.

A CIP catalogue record for this book
is available from the British Library.

ISBN 978-0-349-40981-8

Text design by Laura K. Corless
Printed and bound in Great Britain by
Clays Ltd, St Ives plc

Papers used by Piatkus are from well-managed forests
and other responsible sources.

MIX
Paper from
responsible sources
FSC
www.fsc.org   FSC® C104740

Piatkus
An imprint of
Little, Brown Book Group
Carmelite House
50 Victoria Embankment
London EC4Y 0DZ

An Hachette UK Company
www.hachette.co.uk

www.littlebrown.co.uk

CONTENTS

A note on the client examples presented here:

Client examples included in this book are composites of multiple clients, and details have been changed to protect people's privacy. References to my clinical practice are based on my work in New Zealand from 2008 to 2013.

Disclaimer:

The content of this book is intended for general information purposes only and not as a substitute for individual therapy. Not all of the advice may be right for you.

PART 1

Understanding Yourself and Your Anxiety

CHAPTER 1

. . . .

How Anxiety Works

Does any of this sound familiar?

- You overthink before taking action.
- You're prone to making negative predictions.
- You worry about the worst that could happen.
- You take negative feedback very hard.
- You're self-critical.
- Anything less than extraordinary performance feels like failure.

If yes, you're not alone, and you're probably suffering from some degree of anxiety. Anxiety is an emotional state characterized by feelings of worry, nervousness, and unease. Anxiety disorders affect 40 million Americans over the age of 18, and "everyday anxiety" affects a far greater number.[1]

Based on research, we know that similar psychological mechanisms underlie all types and degrees of anxiety, even if forms of anxiety can look very different on the surface. No matter how your anxiety manifests itself, you'll find the information you're about to read relevant and useful, whether you have an anxiety disorder or are, like me, just anxiety-prone by nature.

....

How Anxiety Works

Anxiety shows up as a variety of symptoms, from behavioral and emotional to physical and cognitive (which just means thoughts). No anxious person has the exact same set of symptoms, but everyone has some of each type. See the table on the next page for examples of each component.

Although anxiety can sometimes seem like a flaw, it's actually an evolutionary advantage, a hypervigilance system that causes us to pause and scan the environment. Feeling anxious triggers us to start looking out for potential threats. If you detect a potential danger, it's not supposed to be easy for you to stop thinking about that threat. While that's great when you're a caveman worried about protecting your family, it's not as great when you're an employee convinced you're getting fired.

For many of us who suffer from anxiety, our anxiety alarms fire too often when there isn't a good reason to be excessively cautious. Why does this happen? We may have more sensitive anxiety systems. Or we may have been doing things to decrease

The Four Components of Anxiety	Examples
Behavioral component	• The urge to put off important but anxiety-provoking tasks • The urge to keep seeking information rather than act • The urge to wait for a go signal from someone else before acting
Emotional component	• Feeling nervous, worried, or apprehensive
Physical component	• Increased heart rate, sick feelings in your stomach
Thought component	• Fear of failure • Mentally replaying events when you're worried about how other people might have perceived you

our anxiety in the short term, such as avoiding things that make us feel anxious, that have actually increased it in the long term.

Having some false anxiety alarms—where you see threats that don't exist or worry about things that don't eventuate—isn't a defect in your system. Think of it in caveman terms: In a life-and-death sense, failing to notice a real threat (termed a *false negative*) is more of a problem than registering a potential danger that doesn't happen (termed a *false positive*). Therefore, having some false anxiety alarms is a built-in part of the system, to err on the side of caution.

People feel anxious when they step outside their comfort zone.

Avoiding stepping outside your comfort zone would lead to living life less fully. Since I'm anxiety-prone by nature, almost every major decision I've made in my life has involved feeling physically sick with anxiety. If I weren't willing to make decisions that lead to temporarily feeling more anxious, my life would be much emptier than it is today.

Reducing your anxiety to zero isn't possible or useful. Anxiety itself isn't the problem. The problem occurs when anxiety gets to the point that it's paralyzing, and you become stuck. I think of these bottlenecks as anxiety traps. We're going to work on managing your responses to five anxiety traps: excessively hesitating before taking action, ruminating and worrying, paralyzing perfectionism, fear of feedback and criticism, and avoidance (including procrastination).

The reason I've chosen to focus on these particular five traps is that I've found them to be the common threads that affect virtually all of the anxious clients I've worked with. The traps are self-perpetuating because they generate additional stress. For example, someone hesitates so much that she misses important opportunities, and this leads to being financially worse off. Or someone avoids feedback and then isn't alerted to real problems that could have been rectified earlier. When people are caught in any of the five anxiety traps, they often fail to see the big picture and don't problem-solve in effective ways. Learning how to navigate these bottlenecks will allow you to manage your anxious tendencies so that you can pursue your goals in life, whatever those goals may be.

How will this book help you learn to successfully navigate your anxiety stuck points? The tools presented here are based on the principles of cognitive behavioral therapy (CBT). CBT is widely regarded as the most effective type of treatment for anxiety and has decades of research behind it.[2] The term *cognitive behavioral* just means that the approach focuses on both thoughts and behaviors and emphasizes that this dual focus is the best way to get results. It's more accurate to say *cognitive behavioral therapies*, since the term actually refers to a family of therapies that have the same underlying principles. However, most people just say "cognitive behavioral therapy," and I'll use the terms interchangeably for convenience.

There are three main things you'll need to successfully navigate your anxiety bottlenecks. The first is self-knowledge about the thinking and behavioral patterns that have caused your anxiety to develop and persist. We know what these are from research on anxiety, and I will discuss how you can learn to recognize them.

The second essential element is a set of tools for coping when you find yourself caught in the web of anxiety. I'll share a toolkit of strategies that will help you unblock your anxiety bottlenecks, so you can head toward your goals and feel better.

The third piece of the puzzle is some general confidence in yourself. You'll need to believe you have the capacity to use the information and tools provided to solve your own problems. If you don't have this self-belief just yet, we'll work on it together—particularly in Part 3.

. . . .

Why This Book Is Different

You may be wondering if this is going to be one of those saccha-rine, stick-a-smiley-face-on-it, positive-thinking books. Heck no. The traditional "Don't worry, be happy" message rubs me the wrong way because I like to feel prepared for things that could go wrong. And I know a lot of other anxious-by-nature people who feel the same way. Many anxious people have had a lifetime of people telling them "Don't worry," "Don't stress," "Don't over-think it." As a result of constantly being told to just relax more and chill out, anxious people often end up feeling like there is something fundamentally wrong with their natural self. The "Don't worry, be happy" message ignores research showing that there are benefits to both optimism and what's termed *defensive pessimism*.[3]

Successfully navigating anxiety involves learning how to ac-cept, like, and work with your nature rather than fighting against it. Personally, I like my nature, even though I'm anxiety-prone. If you don't already, I hope you'll come to understand and like your natural self too. Once anxiety isn't impeding you, this will be easier to accomplish. If you take nothing else away from this book, understand that there's nothing wrong with having a pre-disposition to anxiety. It's fine to be someone who likes to mull things over and consider things that could go wrong. If you're not spontaneous or happy-go-lucky by nature, there's absolutely *nothing* wrong with that either. It's fine to consider potential negative outcomes . . . as long as you also:

- Consider potential positive outcomes.
- Recognize that a *possible* negative outcome isn't necessarily a reason not to do something.
- Recognize your innate capacity to cope with things that don't go according to plan.

In the coming chapters, you'll learn some tips and tricks for switching out of anxiety mode when the volume gets turned up too high. You can use these micro-interventions to handle times when you find yourself overchecking, overresearching, overthinking, or being unwilling to try something that's important to you because of the chance that something might go wrong. You don't need to fundamentally change your nature; you just need to understand your thinking style and learn tricks so you can shift your thoughts and behavior when it's advantageous to *you* to do so.

Another way this book differs? I've learned from the adults I've worked with that they want to understand the principles behind the advice they're being sold. They want to adapt specific strategies to suit their personality, their lifestyle, and their goals. This book will give you the tools and encouragement to do that. I'm going to help you navigate, but ultimately you are the driver.

....

How Did I End Up Writing This Book?

Even though I don't have an anxiety disorder, I've always been anxiety-prone. I was the type of kid who refused to go to camp because I was terrified that the camp leaders would make me eat food I didn't like or tell me off for something I hadn't meant to do. In the days leading up to a new school year, I would get so stressed out about having to adjust to a new teacher that I'd feel physically sick.

Before I started graduate school, I had very little understanding of my own anxiety. I then trained in clinical psychology, which is the psychology of treating disorders, like panic disorder, obsessive-compulsive disorder, depression, and eating disorders. During my training in cognitive behavioral therapies, I noticed how much CBT was helping me understand my own thinking and behavioral patterns. I wasn't using the exact techniques used to treat clients with clinical problems, but I used the principles I was learning to change my thinking patterns and ways of reacting to stress.

When I graduated and started my own practice, I found that the initial problems people came to see me for would often resolve relatively quickly using a CBT approach. For example, when people came for treatment of panic attacks, they would often stop having panic attacks quite quickly. If they came for depression, their mood would frequently lift quickly to the point they wouldn't be considered clinically depressed anymore. When people came for problems with binge eating, they would often break the cycle of bingeing and dieting after just a few weeks of treatment. These people weren't problem-free at this point—they just weren't showing their main symptoms anymore. They still had a lot of questions about how to cope with anxiety and stress and needed additional skills for doing this. The therapies I'd learned didn't seem as useful for this stage of the treatment process, so I started developing my own materials. I was guided by my clients, by research findings, and by what I know works for me in terms of coping with life and anxiety.

I began sharing the materials I'd developed on a blog, and was soon approached by magazines to give expert tips for their stories. I found there was a lot of interest in learning how to use cognitive behavioral tools to solve everyday problems. This interest often came from people who struggled with a degree of anxiety but didn't have clinical disorders. I also noticed that people who had anxiety disorders would come to see me for treatment based on information I'd written on my blog or in magazine articles. The information they were finding useful was about general cognitive behavioral principles but wasn't necessarily specific to their disorder.

As my career progressed, I began to specialize in adapting CBT principles into tools that can be used for dealing with everyday problems, especially anxiety. Because I trained in both clinical and social psychology, I am able to incorporate knowledge from both areas. As a result, my approach is a bit different from other people's. I'm able to blend information from social psychology research (about how people generally think and behave) with that of clinical psychology.

The tools you'll learn about have not only worked for me but have also worked for my clients, and I hope they'll work for you too. I continue to use virtually all of the principles I'm going to share with you. Because it's been more than 10 years since I started my training in CBT and because I use the principles and tools every day, I now use extreme shortcut versions of the tools themselves. The more you practice, the more you'll develop your own shortcuts.

....

What's Coming Next

This book is divided into three parts. Part 1 lays the groundwork for you to understand how anxiety works and better understand your nature. In Part 2, each chapter deals with a specific anxiety bottleneck. For each bottleneck, I'll provide you with a toolkit of actionable strategies to unblock it. In Part 3, we'll cover how to integrate the material into your life going forward and proactively troubleshoot problems that people often encounter. I'll also offer suggestions for ongoing self-development work that goes beyond the anxiety focus of this book.

From this point onward, each chapter in the book begins with a quiz so that you can gauge how relevant that particular chapter is likely to be for you and get a sense of the learning aims for the chapter. Each quiz question requires you to answer A, B, C, or (sometimes) D. The content of the chapter will help you move toward the A answers.

Within each of the chapters in Part 2, we'll cover recommended thinking shifts and then behavioral shifts. For each thinking shift, there will be a thought experiment to help you make the change. You'll probably want to keep a notebook handy while you read for completing these experiments.

. . . .

Use This Book in the Way That Works Best for You

You can interact with the material I'm sharing however is best for you. Remember: You're aiming to build your own personalized Anxiety Toolkit by finding strategies you like and adapting them to suit yourself.

Here are a few things to keep in mind:

This book is intended as a reference book. You can dip back into any chapter as required. Come back to the material when you need to get insight into a problem you're having or when you want to try something new (like when you're in the mood to try a new recipe). If you start to feel a sense of information overload, stop reading once you've gained an insight that you want to implement in your life. You can always come back to the rest of the material whenever you feel like it.

You may notice that thinking and reading about anxiety causes you to feel some of your anxiety symptoms. The times when this happens can be a bit random. If it happens one day, it won't necessarily happen the next time you pick up the book. To be honest, there are times when writing or talking about anxiety triggers anxious feelings for me. This is all par for the course, a course we'll be navigating together. If reading about anxiety is making you anxious at any point, you can choose whether to keep reading and see if it naturally subsides or put the book aside for a few days.

You also may find reading to be a more comfortable state than doing. You may find yourself reluctant to try the suggested experiments because you're not 100% sure if they'll work for you or if you'll do them perfectly. The key is to realize that you can't wait for those feelings and concerns to go away before giving things a go. You'd likely be waiting forever. The good news: Taking any action while feeling a sense of uncertainty will make it easier to take action the next time you're feeling uncertain. Focus on what feels doable, even if that's just a few bits and pieces.

Many people with anxiety have problems with more than one type of anxiety—for example, problems with worry and social anxiety. If this is you, then you're likely to find the *transdiagnostic* (that is, not disorder-specific) approach this book takes particularly useful. If you think you may have a clinical anxiety problem, like social anxiety disorder or panic disorder, then you're likely to benefit from, at some stage, working through a treatment package that's specifically tailored to the problem you have (see TheAnxietyToolkit.com/resources for some suggestions). However, the material in this book will complement that work.

Lastly, sometimes good general advice isn't good advice for *you*. Part of learning to like and accept your nature is empowering yourself to ignore advice that doesn't gel with you. Here's an example: Long before I considered writing a book of my own, I started going to see authors on their book tours. At virtually all these talks, someone in the audience asks the author about his or her writing process. Most authors say they get up at the crack of dawn because they need uninterrupted writing time before their children get up or before they go to their day job. However, at one recent discussion, an author said he writes in little snatches of time throughout the day, whenever he gets an idea—often while he's at work. This sent a hush over the room because it didn't fit the accepted wisdom or the advice the other authors on the panel had given. However, this author had clearly learned to understand his own nature and to ignore advice that didn't work for him.

If you find yourself feeling unwilling to try something in this book, move on from that section. Find something you feel willing to try and start there. Find what works for you based on your preferences and the stage you're at. If you try suggestions and they fizzle, or some of the advice doesn't work for you, feel free to ignore it. That's simply part of beginning to accept your nature. Let's continue to work on that now.

CHAPTER 2

. . . .

Understanding the Multidimensional You

This chapter introduces some core personality and wiring concepts that will help you understand how your mind works. Awareness of these aspects of your nature will help you better understand your anxiety.

Take the following quiz to see how this chapter pertains to you. Choose the answer that *best* applies. If no answer is the perfect fit, pick whichever is the closest.

1. How well do you understand your fundamental nature?

(A) I have a good understanding of what motivates me and what causes me to feel emotionally balanced or unbalanced.

(B) There are some aspects of myself I don't understand.

(C) There are many aspects of myself I don't understand.

2. Do you ever feel like your natural instincts are in conflict? For example, you want to reach for new opportunities, but then your instinct to worry about what might go wrong kicks in and you freeze up.

   (A) I can keep a balance between being focused on potential rewards and worrying about things that could go wrong.

   (B) Sometimes.

   (C) Yes, this gets in my way a great deal.

3. How well do you understand what tends to overstimulate you? For example, too much social contact or abrupt changes of plans.

   (A) I understand what leaves me feeling jangled. My life is set up to minimize these occurrences and to allow me to effectively reset when I do get overstimulated.

   (B) I'd like to understand this better.

   (C) I haven't thought about this.

4. Are you able to distinguish between conscientiousness and perfectionism?

   (A) Yes, I recognize how striving for perfection can sometimes result in being less conscientious overall.

   (B) Theoretically yes, but in practice I frequently confuse the two.

   (C) They seem like the same thing to me.

5. **How easily are you able to recognize useful types of care and caution vs. times when care and caution become paralyzing?**

   (A) I can see when being careful and cautious is an asset and when it isn't, and can adjust my behavior accordingly.

   (B) Sometimes I realize that I'm being too careful or cautious, but I seem to have no control over it.

   (C) If I'm being excessively careful or cautious, I usually don't notice this until long after the fact, if at all.

6. **How easily are you able to moderate aspects of your nature? For example, if you're very persistent, can you moderate your behavior in instances when taking a break is a better idea than continuing to bang your head against a problem?**

   (A) Most of the time.

   (B) I'm hit or miss at this.

   (C) No.

Here's how to interpret your scores. If you scored:

Mostly A's

You understand yourself well and can moderate any strong tendencies you have so that they work to your advantage and don't cause problems for you. While you may not need all the information in this chapter, there's likely to be at least one or two nuggets of useful info for you here.

Mostly B's

You understand yourself to some degree but sometimes have difficulty moderating dominant tendencies that might not be the best match for a particular situation. This chapter offers you the opportunity to develop an even more advanced and nuanced understanding of what makes you tick.

Mostly C's

You may recognize there are ways you seem different from other people, but you feel either confused or ashamed about these. This chapter will help you better understand your nature and how you can best work with it to minimize excessive anxiety. The chapter will also help you recognize times when you get caught up in counterproductive types of care and caution.

To better manage your anxiety, you don't need to understand the average anxious person—you need to understand the multidimensional you. By *multidimensional*, I mean understanding your nature beyond just your predisposition to anxiety. For example, someone who is anxious and agreeable will be different from someone who is anxious and disagreeable. Very agreeable individuals might react to anxiety by agreeing to things they feel uncomfortable with. Disagreeable people might react to anxiety by nitpicking others' ideas or seeing only the flaws in plans, leading them to opt out of potentially exciting collaborations.

Because a variety of traits shape anyone's individual thinking and motivational style, not just anxiety, it's important that I briefly introduce some core wiring concepts, which will help you understand how you tick. I can't cover everything, but these are some of the areas of personality and temperament that I end up talking about most often with anxiety-prone people. Understanding these concepts will help you gain the broad-ranging self-knowledge you'll need to figure yourself out, discover your optimal way of operating, and increase your sense of positive self-acceptance. Not every section of this chapter will be relevant for every reader, but if a section isn't relevant for you personally, it will help you understand other people.

············

Introversion and Extraversion

The stereotype of an anxious person tends to be synonymous with that of an introvert. There is some truth to this perception in that, statistically, people with anxiety disorders are more likely to be introverts.[1] However, some of the clients I've seen who have struggled the most with anxiety have been extraverts.

For example, in some ways, social anxiety is an easier affliction for an introvert to deal with. If socially anxious introverts can work around their social anxiety enough to form a few close relationships in which they don't feel anxious anymore, they can often feel OK. The socially anxious extravert craves more than a small inner circle of confidants and loved ones.

If you're an anxious extravert, acknowledge your extraversion and that it's normal (even if somewhat less common) for extraversion to coexist with anxiety. As we proceed, I'll help you understand the psychology behind why your anxiety causes you to hold back from the social interaction you crave and prevents you from being true to your fundamental nature as an extravert. Once you understand why you're holding back, you'll be able to use cognitive behavioral tools to overcome those psychological barriers.

. . . .

The Highly Sensitive Person

Sometimes qualities that get lumped together as part of introversion or anxiety are more closely related to a concept known in psychology as *high sensitivity*.[2] Some of the typical characteristics of a highly sensitive person (HSP) include tendencies to:

- Process things deeply
- Get easily overwhelmed by too many things to do
- Get their feelings hurt easily
- Be sensitive to other people's moods
- Find negative news very upsetting, even if it's about people they don't know well
- Find it difficult to hide their true feelings, such as when they lack interest in a topic
- Find it difficult to filter out particular types of stimulation, such as being easily irritated by background noise or scratchy textured clothing

People who have a lot of these tendencies aren't necessarily anxious. However, they will often become anxious if they're forced into environments that overwhelm their capacity to filter excess stimulation. For example, I had a client with symptoms that were a lot like depression and anxiety. This normally happy person felt tearful frequently, was unable to focus, and was irritable all the time. Together we figured out that the problem was due to her company switching her to an open-plan office. She couldn't filter out all the excess stimulation created by that change in her work space. This is a great example of how you need to understand your nature to understand your anxiety and mood. If you think you might be an HSP, I recommend you read Dr. Elaine Aron's book, *The Highly Sensitive Person*, alongside this book.[3] Like any book, take what you find useful from it and ignore the rest.

....

Prevention vs. Promotion Focus

Anxiety is often associated with having a *prevention focus*.[4] This means being focused on preventing bad things from happening. In contrast, *promotion focus* means being focused on reaching for new opportunities and rewards. While most people have a dominant focus, it's possible to be high in both types, meaning you're naturally very concerned both with avoiding mistakes and harm and with reaching for opportunities. This can result in a constant sense of pushing forward and pulling back.

Sometimes the association between anxiety and prevention

focus is extrapolated to suggest that anxious people might be most suited to jobs and careers where being conservative, being careful, and maintaining the status quo are the top priorities. In my experience working with clients, these types of careers can sometimes make things worse for highly anxious people. For example, medical doctors are encouraged to be very thorough and careful. For doctors, it's constantly (and rightly) reinforced that not being extremely careful could have disastrous consequences. However, for people who are already worriers, this focus on the need to be careful at all times in the workplace can sometimes worsen their general tendencies to worry and check excessively.

I've also seen this happen to people in other careers where attention to detail is highly valued and rewarded, such as graphic design. Being in a career where "sweating the small stuff" is encouraged sometimes causes this to spill over into people's personal lives. If you're in this situation, you don't need to change careers; you just need to recognize and understand how the principles that help you succeed at work might not apply in every situation.

. . . .

Sensation Seeking

If you've got anxious tendencies, but the thought of being in a job where the main focus is on avoiding mistakes seems boring to you, you might be someone who is high in what's called *sensation seeking*. Being high in sensation seeking involves enjoying an element of risk and craving novelty. If you're high in both sensation seeking and sensitivity, it may feel as if you are walking a tightrope between doing things that excite you and not getting wiped out by the stimulation that comes along with novelty.

If all these terms seem confusing, it's because researchers working in different areas of psychology use their own terms to describe overlapping (but different) concepts. You don't need to worry too much about nuances. The take-home message is that there are people who are ambitious, competitive, big thinking, and novelty seeking, who have other elements of their nature that can cause them to get easily overstimulated or to slam on their brakes when their instinct to be cautious kicks in. People who have these seemingly competing tendencies will likely benefit a great deal from the material in this book. When your nature is a bit complex, having a manual to figure it out helps.

. . . .

Processing Change

One of the ways people fundamentally differ from one another is that individuals vary in how much emotional energy it takes for them to process change or the idea of change. For example, some people may find it incredibly jarring when they have to deal with last-minute changes in plans or they have to work with different people from those they usually work with. People who need time and psychological space to adjust to change won't necessarily be anxious. However, they'll tend to develop anxiety if they aren't allowed, or don't allow themselves, the time they need to adjust to change, or if they don't have any emotional energy in their tank to cope with small changes in plans.

Are folks who require more energy to process change always rigid and unadaptable? No. They can still be very good at adapting—if they have the self-knowledge to navigate changes in a way that works for their nature. They will generally function best if they have habits, routines, and relationships in their life that give them a base level of consistency and familiarity. This could be as simple as eating the same thing for breakfast every day, having stable long-term relationships, or having particular routines for what they like to do on the weekend. Having some stable, familiar elements to life can help people tolerate changes in other areas.

Of note, you can be someone who finds change exciting (that is, a sensation seeker) but also finds it psychologically taxing. Human nature is complicated!

. . . .

The Agreeable vs. the Disagreeable Anxious Person

Earlier I mentioned people being agreeable or disagreeable. Being generally agreeable or disagreeable has been identified as one of the fundamental dimensions of personality.[5] Just like anyone else, anxious people can be either agreeable or disagreeable. It pays to know which you are. People who are agreeable tend to prioritize getting along with others. They may not be willing to make waves when they can see problems with other people's ideas or plans. In contrast, people who are naturally disagreeable may underestimate the importance of getting along with others and not invest enough in relationship building.[6]

Once you can recognize whatever tendencies you have, you can keep them in mind and modify your responses as you see fit. For example, if you're anxious and disagreeable, you may say no more than you should. After all, your nature has you on the lookout for things that could go wrong. My mom often refers to my stepdad and me as people who "start at no and might move to yes." She's someone who's highly agreeable and therefore automatically starts at yes and only very rarely moves to no.

If you're anxious and agreeable, you may find yourself overcommitting to things because you overestimate the potential negative consequences of saying no. More generally, you may hold back from saying things you want to say because of anxiety about how you'll be perceived. The skills you'll learn in this book will help you balance your goal of being well liked with other priorities—like managing your schedule and speaking your mind.

Whether you're naturally agreeable or disagreeable, you can stay true to your general nature but develop the ability to switch out of that mindset when it's creating a bias or causing problems in your relationships.

....

Conscientiousness

Not every anxious person is conscientious, but because you're reading a CBT-based self-help book, there's a good chance you're at least moderately high in conscientiousness—a personality trait associated with having a strong work ethic and a thorough, orderly approach to tasks. People high in conscientiousness often get particularly great results from learning cognitive behavioral principles and skills. Why? They tend to like the systematic nature of a cognitive behavioral approach. They do well because they work hard to understand themselves and are diligent in applying their learning to their lives. Anxious people sometimes underestimate how conscientious they are, so make sure you give yourself enough credit for your conscientiousness.

It's important to understand that conscientiousness is not the same thing as perfectionism. For example, perfectionists might spend so long trying to make something "just right" that they don't have any willpower left over for other important tasks. Perfectionism and conscientiousness tend to be associated with opposite outcomes. For example, in a study of older adults, perfectionism was associated with an increased risk of mortality. Conscientiousness was associated with a decreased risk.[7] There are big advantages to reducing perfectionism but retaining your conscientiousness!

Many of the tools you'll learn in this book will help you turn down the volume on counterproductive types of perfectionism, including an entire chapter devoted just to this (Chapter 6). For now, the two exercises that follow will help you distinguish between useful and not useful types of care and caution and how these are linked to anxiety.

Useful Types of Care and Caution

I'm going to give you some examples of how anxiety can motivate useful types of care and caution. When you understand that the adaptive function of anxiety is to put you on the lookout for danger, you can begin to recognize how having a predisposition to anxiety can potentially benefit you if you channel it in the right direction.

Experiment: In the chart that follows, you'll find the general principle in the left-hand column and my examples in the right-hand column. I'm going to share my own examples from time to time throughout this book to keep things real and to avoid breaking client confidentiality by sharing other people's examples that are too specific.

Where you can relate to the principles, try coming up with your own examples. Some people go into freeze mode when they're asked to think of examples. If this is you, that's OK—just read mine.

Examples of Having an Anxious Nature	Examples of How Conscientiousness, Care, and Caution Can Be Productive
When I make plans, I think about possible things that could go wrong. I make contingency plans.	• I take an extra credit card when going on an overseas trip in case my main card isn't working for some reason.
When something going wrong seems likely, I take precautions to minimize any potential harm.	• I keep receipts for things I might need to return. • If a customer service person tells me something on the phone and I'm concerned the person is giving me the wrong info, I'll ask the agent to note what I was told on my account and read back to me what was written. I'll also ask for the person's agent ID number.
I'm extremely thorough when I do research.	• I'm *not* the type of person who arrives at a beach vacation only to find it's the middle of monsoon season.
Being anxious about looking good in the eyes of others causes me to be polite and to prepare thoroughly.	• I'll generally jot down a few brief notes or questions before a meeting. • I write notes in meetings so that the person I'm speaking with recognizes that I value what he or she is saying.
I do things carefully.	• I have routines for doing things, so I don't lose keys or accidentally leave the stove on.
I think things over before making decisions.	• When I need to make a purchase, I'll usually research online before visiting a store. Up to a point, I enjoy this. It saves me time returning purchases made on impulse.
Because I'm on the lookout for problems, I'm less vulnerable to being taken advantage of.	• When I know I'll be needing to take a cab in a foreign country, I find out what the approximate price should be beforehand.

Counterproductive Types of Care and Caution

The same careful and cautious tendencies that can be helpful in some situations can become paralyzing in others. You might hold back from opportunities or get caught up in minutia while leaving bigger issues unattended. Very cautious tendencies can also cause people to hold back from attempting to form relationships—whether they be friendships or romantic, business, or collegial relationships. There's always some level of vulnerability that comes along with developing any type of close relationship. Therefore, in some cases, anxiety-based instincts to be self-protective can leave people feeling isolated and alone. Anxious people will sometimes avoid feeling vulnerable at all costs, even if it means feeling lonely or their isolation from peers thwarts their career success.

Experiment: The list of principles in the following table is the same as in the first experiment. This time I've included my examples of how these same tendencies can become *unhelpful*. Although I manage to avoid falling into these traps most of the time, I still find myself caught in them occasionally. If you can relate, think about or write down a few of your own examples. You could also just put a check mark in the right-hand column, where applicable, to indicate "That's me."

Examples of Having an Anxious Nature	Examples of How Care and Caution Can Be Counterproductive
When I make plans, I think about possible things that could go wrong. I make contingency plans.	• I sometimes find myself unwilling to try things because of the potential for something to go wrong.
When something seems likely to go wrong, I take precautions to minimize any potential harm.	• I sometimes spend so much time trying to prevent things from going wrong in unimportant areas that I run out of time and willpower to do it in more important areas.
I'm extremely thorough when I do research.	• I sometimes get stuck in research mode for long periods.
Being anxious about looking good in the eyes of others causes me to be polite and to prepare thoroughly.	• Sometimes I get so anxious about how I'm perceived that I try to control how others perceive me. I act controlling or end up mentally replaying conversations, wondering if I said the right thing. • Being anxious about how others perceive me sometimes causes me to jump to the conclusion that other people don't like me, when that's not the reality. Because I perceive that I'm being judged negatively, I act less open/friendly and sometimes create a self-fulfilling prophecy.
I do things carefully.	• Sometimes I'll spend ridiculously excessive amounts of time on tasks. • I sometimes find myself overchecking some things and ignoring other work that's objectively a higher priority.
I think things over before making decisions.	• I sometimes spend hours overthinking a $100 decision when I could've put that time toward something that would've generated two or three times that amount in income.

Examples of Having an Anxious Nature	Examples of How Care and Caution Can Be Counterproductive
Because I'm on the lookout for problems, I'm less vulnerable to being taken advantage of.	• I'm sometimes excessively suspicious of other people, to the point where I avoid collaborations.

. . . .

Moderating Your Thinking Style and Behaviors

Strong personality traits can sometimes give you a huge competitive advantage over other people—they can help you achieve things others don't. However, the trick is moderating these personality traits so that they don't dominate your nature. For example, being extremely persistent—which anxious, high achievers often are—can have a huge upside. However, if you're very persistent but can't moderate it, it can be difficult to take a break in situations in which you need one. You might find it hard to step away when you're stuck on a task and not getting anywhere or when you're involved in an argument that's going nowhere and only getting more heated. The more extreme a trait is, the more likely it is to be a double-edged sword—sometimes useful and sometimes not.

So far, we've been working on you developing a nuanced understanding of your patterns. As you move through this book, you'll learn ways of moderating the less-than-helpful patterns you've identified while retaining the elements that are useful to you and that help you feel like you're being true to your nature.

CHAPTER 3

....

Your Goals

One of the ways severe anxiety sucks people into its vortex is that avoiding anxiety often becomes the person's central focus. The more this happens, the more anxious the person becomes. When people overfocus on anxiety for a long time, they tend to lose confidence in their capacity to be anything other than a walking ball of worry and rumination. This chapter will help you connect with your non-anxiety-related goals, so you have something you can move toward while you are also moving away from excessive anxiety.

Take the following quiz to see how this chapter pertains to you. Choose the answer that *best* applies. If no answer is the perfect fit, pick whichever is the closest.

1. **Do you ever worry that you're weak or crazy because your anxiety has gotten out of control?**

   (A) Neither of these.

   (B) One of these.

   (C) How did you know? Both of these.

2. **Do you ever find yourself overmonitoring your symptoms of anxiety?**

   (A) No.

   (B) Rarely.

   (C) Yes. I monitor my anxiety like it's a weather report.

3. **Do you avoid pursuing some of your goals and dreams due to anxiety?**

   (A) No. Although anxiety is unpleasant, achieving my goals and dreams is worth tolerating any anxiety I might experience along the way.

   (B) There are a few goals or dreams I don't pursue because of anxiety, even though I'd like to.

   (C) When I'm reading *O* magazine in the supermarket checkout line and I see "living your best life" mentioned, my heart sinks because I know I'm not living mine.

4. **How easy or difficult is it for you to identify personal goals that might seem unimportant to others but that feel very meaningful to you?**

   (A) I have a good sense of who I am and what my interests are. It's easy to think of goals and dreams that reflect this.

   (B) I can think of some quirky goals, but I'd feel too embarrassed or unsure of myself to pursue them.

   (C) I feel disconnected from knowing who I am. This makes it difficult to identify my unique goals and dreams.

5. **Does your self-esteem come from multiple spheres of your life or is it concentrated in one or two domains (for example, your looks, your career success, or your role as a parent)?**

   (A) My self-esteem comes from a variety of sources: everything from the fact that I recycle to the fact that my friends ask for seconds when I serve them my massaman curry.

   (B) Over 85% of my self-esteem comes from only two domains.

   (C) Over 85% of my self-esteem comes from a single domain.

6. **Are you willing to tolerate feelings of vulnerability?**

   (A) Yes, I pursue things that feel meaningful, even when this involves tolerating a sense of vulnerability.

(B) I find it hard to tolerate feeling vulnerable and usually avoid situations that provoke this.

(C) Even hearing the word *vulnerable* makes me feel like running for the hills. Eliminating stress and other unpleasant emotions is my main focus.

Here's how to interpret your scores. If you scored:

Mostly A's

Although anxiety is part of your life, you don't shy away from your goals and dreams because of it. You know yourself well, and your goals are like a mirror that reflects the core of who you are. You recognize that pursuing things that provide meaning in life involves experiencing a few anxiety jitters. You believe in your capacity to cope with that. Your self-esteem is diversified rather than hinging on only one area of your life. This diversification helps provide a psychological buffer when things aren't going according to plan in one area. Expect to be able to move quickly through this chapter.

Mostly B's

You've lost confidence in your ability to pursue some of your goals and dreams but not to the extent that all your goals are on pause. This chapter will help you understand the psychological mechanisms of how, as anxiety increases, life tends to shrink. You'll also learn how to reverse this pattern.

Mostly C's

Avoiding anxiety has become a major focus of your life, to the point that other goals have faded into the background. You've lost confidence in yourself. You likely have a sense that anxiety has taken over your life. This chapter will help you understand the psychological processes that cause anxiety to snowball and how you can rediscover goals and dreams beyond just your goal of reducing anxiety.

The more time and energy people spend managing their anxiety, the more it sucks the oxygen out of the rest of their life. In this chapter, I'll explain how focusing on your anxiety causes it to escalate. You'll then learn how reducing your anxiety requires discovering or rediscovering goals that are more important to you than avoiding anxiety. I'll show you how you can reconnect with your goals and increase your resiliency.

Let's unpack the psychological mechanisms of how anxiety snowballs.

· · · · · · · · · · · · ·

Trying to Eliminate Anxiety Can Cause More Anxiety

When anxiety becomes a major problem for someone, it's usually because the person has become stuck in a self-perpetuating cycle where the things he or she does to reduce anxiety in the short term cause it to multiply in the long term. Let me explain how this works.

Let's take someone who gets panic attacks. Because these are so unpleasant, the person logically avoids situations that might trigger an attack. The person might start out avoiding a few situations, such as public speaking or going to the mall on weekends. Paradoxically, the more the person avoids particular situations, the more their anxiety about having another panic attack increases. An increasing number of situations start to trigger their anxiety. The person starts to avoid more and more. The problem snowballs. Avoiding things due to anxiety is termed *avoidance coping*. It's one of the main mechanisms that causes anxiety to grow and persist. It's a theme we'll return to repeatedly, especially in Chapter 8, which is devoted to overcoming avoidance.

Let's work through another example: People with eating disorders fear gaining weight, so they cut out more and more foods. They might start out avoiding butter. This helps them feel better temporarily, but soon other types of foods start to make them feel anxious about gaining weight. They start avoiding those too. The cycle continues, and they might end up eating only rice crackers and celery sticks. The more foods they avoid, the worse their anxiety about food usually gets. When they get to the point that eating a normal meal feels utterly terrifying, they usually start to think they're losing their mind. (Yes, even people with severe eating disorders know that being more worried about the fat grams in an avocado than about global warming is a little off-kilter.)

"Hey, Alice, isn't this a book about anxiety? Why are you bringing up eating disorders?" Great question. I'm mentioning eating disorders to show that common mental health issues that look quite different on the surface—and even those that aren't necessarily classified as anxiety problems, such as eating disorders and depression—often have similar underlying psychological mechanisms. This is part of the reason I can confidently say that the tips in this book will apply to people with a wide range of anxiety-related issues.

Let's consider a less severe example: Bridget feels anxious about fixing the computer and emailing the accountant so she asks her partner, Steve, to do these things for her. The more people rely on their loved ones to do things for them when they feel anxious, the more their anxiety is likely to grow. Over time, they will feel less and less competent. They'll increasingly doubt their ability to cope with situations that provoke anxiety. More and more situations will set off their self-doubt. Their relationships are also likely to suffer.

People often develop routines or rituals to try to keep a lid on their anxiety. These can range from avoiding "forbidden foods," to going to only certain places or doing only certain activities with someone else, to washing their hands for a minimum number of seconds. Again, these routines help relieve anxiety in the short term but increase it in the long term, and suck away self-confidence. The good news is that cognitive behavioral strategies are very effective for preventing anxiety from spiraling out of control and for reversing this process once it has occurred.

· · · · · · · · · · · ·

Labeling Yourself as Crazy or Weak

When anxiety has become severe, people often go from seeing themselves as "normal" or at least normal*ish*, to wondering if they're crazy. If your anxiety has led you to this point, don't despair. This is just what happens when people get stuck in the anxiety catch-22: You avoid things that make you feel anxious, but then end up more anxious overall. When you stop doing the things that are causing your anxiety to grow (which this book will help you with), you'll start to feel like your mind belongs to you again.

When people's anxiety is less severe, they might not worry that they're going crazy. Instead, they'll often feel like their anxiety is holding them back. If they're not making as much progress with their goals as they'd like, they'll wonder if they're a fundamentally weak or incompetent person. Some people believe their anxiety makes them broken and unlovable. They might question if they're ever going to have satisfying connections with other people or if they're destined for a life of rejection and loneliness.

· · · · · · · · · · · ·

Overmonitoring

Avoidance coping is one behavioral pattern that causes anxiety to grow like a weed; another is overmonitoring your symptoms. Have you ever found yourself unable to sleep? You end up looking at the clock and counting the minutes you've been lying there tossing and turning. "I've been trying to get to sleep for 40 minutes now!" Another hour passes and you think, "It's two a.m.; now I'm only going to get five hours of sleep before I have to get up for work." The more minutes tick by, the more stressed out you get. The next day, every time you yawn, you worry about getting to sleep that night. Later, when you get into bed, your anxiety about getting to sleep becomes a self-fulfilling prophecy.[1] Sound familiar? It's the natural pattern that happens when you overmonitor something.

This same pattern happens with anxiety symptoms. The more closely individuals monitor their symptoms, the more stressed out by them they become. When people make reducing anxiety their primary focus, they usually do a lot of checking in with themselves about how anxious they feel at any given moment and what anxiety-provoking situations they have coming up. They might wake up in the morning and immediately ask, "How anxious do I feel today?" Overall, this tends to make their anxious feelings worse.

Have you ever had a situation in which focusing on your anxiety symptoms has caused them to increase?

People sometimes think they need to reduce their anxiety before they start thinking about other goals. However, because overfocusing on anxiety isn't helpful, that's the wrong way around. You need to have your goals clearly in mind first, and then think about how you can pursue them without getting derailed by anxiety. Let's turn to that now.

. . . .

Rediscover Your Goals

This section is about connecting with your deepest, most important goals. Your goals don't need to be of the "become so rich I get to hang out with celebrities" variety. Nor do they need an approval stamp from anyone who's not directly involved. What they do need to be is personally meaningful for you.

Find the Goals Where Pursuing Them Is Worth Tolerating Anxiety

If you've got severe anxiety, it may have created a goals vacuum in your life. It may seem like your anxiety problems have been so all-consuming that you haven't focused much on anything else. This is understandable. Since overcoming anxiety involves moving toward something, not just moving away from anxiety, it'll involve rediscovering what your goals are. You need to uncover the goals that genuinely light your fire, where pursuing them is worth tolerating the anxiety that they create. Finding those goals is a very personal process.

Experiment: Can you think of anything that you want more than you fear? Your example could be anything from buying an investment property to taking up jogging (people who are anxious sometimes avoid vigorous exercise because the sensations mimic their physical anxiety symptoms). If you can't think of anything right now, the rest of the chapter might spark your thinking, or you might need to let the question marinate for a few days.

Goals Don't Need to Be Giant to Be Important to You

I often feel tinges of inadequacy when I read business and success books because they seem to be aimed at people who have sky-high goals. It shouldn't be assumed that all of us would want to be a CEO of a huge company or have similarly ambitious goals if only we were more confident and self-assured. Try thinking about your idiosyncratic goals. You might not have any desire to fly first class or have employees. Your goals might be to take a year off to travel, become a TV reviewer for a website, start a podcast, write a book of essays, go to Comic Con, or find meaningful volunteer work. Don't be afraid to acknowledge your idiosyncratic goals, no matter how nerdtastic (or conventional) they seem.

When you're thinking about goals, keep in mind that more ambitious goals aren't "better" than less ambitious goals. Many people would rather visit 30 countries in a lifetime than 200. Many people would rather run a small business than a big business. Many people would rather have a small house than a house that's three times the size they need.

You might not have any plan for how your goals are going to eventuate just yet, but it's still OK to have the goal. For example, one of my idiosyncratic goals was to visit Google—not to work there or start a company as successful as Google but just to go visit. This was not an opportunity I expected to come up anytime soon. However, it did come up when my friend Dr. Guy Winch mentioned he was going to be giving a book talk at its New York campus.[2] At that moment, I needed to decide if I had the gumption to ask if I could tag along. It was either speak up or give in to my anxiety that Guy might perceive my request as weird or inappropriate. What happened? My desire to go won out over my anxiety about making the request. Guy said he was happy for me to go. And yes, the experience completely lived up to expectations!

I'm often amazed at how many of my quirky goals I've achieved. For example, I once went to Starbucks with my favorite Broadway actress. How? Because in an extreme fan-girl moment I asked her, and she agreed. I'm still mortifyingly embarrassed I went through with asking, but despite that embarrassment, it was one of my life highlights! If you feel embarrassed because some of your goals seem off the wall, that's OK.

Experiment: What's one idiosyncratic goal that's important to you? The purpose here is simply to acknowledge the goal to yourself.

Acknowledge When You're Restricting Your Goals Due to Anxiety

As I've said, small goals are just as valid as big goals. However, there are some instances when anxiety causes people to restrict their goals. It's important to acknowledge when this is happening. People with shaky self-worth may hold back from setting ambitious goals because they worry that others will see them as too confident or full of themselves. However, setting less ambitious goals sometimes backfires. For example, people who hold back from thinking big may end up working in ineffective or inefficient ways because they're not as focused on developing scalable systems as they would be if they were thinking bigger.

Sometimes we set lower goals because we "fear success." When people talk about fear of success, they're talking about anticipatory anxiety related to what they predict success would bring. You can confront and problem-solve this fear, but first you need to identify what you're actually anxious about.

Experiment: Are there goals that interest you, but anxiety is causing you to choose smaller targets than you might otherwise? Can you identify specifically what it is you're worried about? For example, you might fear that success will mean drowning in your inbox and other increased social demands. Your worry might be that you won't get the alone time you need to feel balanced. How could you problem-solve this fear? For example, what might you do to cope if greater success meant receiving a lot more email?

What larger targets would you set if you didn't fear success?

Expose Yourself to Opportunity

Achieving personal dreams doesn't always arise out of relentless pursuit of goals. Sometimes you achieve dreams simply by exposing yourself to life. If you're restricting how much you're living your life due to feelings of anxiety, you'll miss out on unexpected opportunities to achieve your goals. Here's an example: A friend of mine had the goal of meeting author Malcolm Gladwell. He was near the top of the list of people she most wanted to meet in her lifetime. She was visiting New York City from New Zealand and found herself sitting across from him in a coffee shop. This was an incredibly lucky coincidence, but it wouldn't have occurred if she'd been sitting at home in New Zealand, rather than sitting in the West Village.

Experiment: Have you ever had the experience of achieving a goal or dream by putting yourself in the right place at the right time? Have you noticed that you expose yourself to less of these opportunities when you're focused on your anxiety?

Embrace Your Nature

As we discussed in the last chapter, how sensation seeking you are is biological and wired into your personality. If you have only a few goals, it could be that your preferences for novelty and intense experiences are on the lower end of the spectrum, not that you lack goals. If you're constantly thinking of new goals, there's nothing wrong with that either. It suggests you're hardwired with a high need for novelty and excitement.

. . . .

Set Goals That Will Build Resiliency

Building resiliency is one way you can prevent yourself from getting derailed by anxiety. *Resiliency* refers to the strengths and resources you have for coping with stress and challenges. All the skills you learn in this book will help you build your resiliency.

Here I'm going to share two ways you can increase your resiliency that relate to the types of goals you choose.

Pursue Meaning, Not Happiness

Feeling happy is like feeling warm. It's a state of being that feels good. It might sound counterintuitive but focusing directly on pursuing happiness isn't always the best approach to increasing it. This parallels the idea that focusing on reducing anxiety isn't always the best way to decrease it.

What's an alternative to focusing on increasing your happiness? A better idea is focusing on pursuing things that feel meaningful. I'm not necessarily suggesting Mother Teresa–type activities. What gives you a sense of meaning could be anything from cooking for your friends to puttering away on projects in your garage.

Pursuing meaning rather than happiness helps you feel calmer when you're not feeling happy in a particular moment. It smooths out the emotional bumps that come with mistakes, failures, and disappointments. There's research showing that stress tends to be harmful only if you believe that it's harmful and that you can't cope with it.[3] It's easier to believe in your capacity to cope with stress if the stress is part of the bigger picture of building a meaningful life.

Experiment: What makes for a meaningful life from your perspective? Skip over what you think you should answer and identify what's actually true for you.

Diversify Your Sources of Self-Esteem

Another way to increase your resiliency is to diversify your sources of self-esteem. Just like putting all your money in a single stock is risky, putting all your self-esteem eggs in one basket is psychologically risky. If your self-esteem is almost entirely based on your career achievements, having a flat stomach, or how hot your boyfriend or girlfriend is, you'll be at more risk of coming unstuck psychologically if your career stalls, you gain weight, or your hot boyfriend or girlfriend dumps you. You'll feel less anxious if your self-esteem isn't too closely tied to just one or two domains.

Experiment: Self-esteem is composed of (1) a sense of self-worth and (2) a sense of being competent at things.[4] For example, sources of self-worth might involve loving and being loved by others; an ability to make other people feel comfortable and at ease; or positive contributions you make to society, your field, or your community. In contrast, a sense of competency might come from being good at computer tasks, being able to prepare a dinner party for 10, or paying your bills on time. Try coming up with three sources of self-worth and three things you're competent at. Aim to recognize areas you've tended to underappreciate.

••••••••••••

Your Goals Will Be Your Compass

Now that you've worked through the chapter, what's on your list of goals that you can definitively say you want to achieve more than you're afraid of attempting? What are you willing to pursue even if you feel anxious and emotionally vulnerable in doing so? The goals you've identified in this chapter are like your compass for the rest of the book. They'll provide you with a sense of direction as you move through the remaining chapters. As you read, keep in mind the idea that you're pursuing goals that have personal meaning for you—that are worth it to you on a deep emotional level—even when the process of pursuing them causes your anxiety to bubble up. Now that we've set a foundation and a direction, we're going to start covering specific anxiety traps. First up: excessive hesitancy when moving from thinking to action.

PART 2

Your Anxiety Toolkit

Overcoming Your Stuck Points

CHAPTER 4

....

Hesitancy

How to Stop Holding Back from the Things You Want to Do

Many anxious people get stuck in thinking mode when they'd really like to give something a go. This is different from putting off things you don't want to do, which we'll cover in Chapter 8. This chapter will help you switch out of contemplation mode and into action mode more easily.

Take the following quiz to see how this chapter pertains to you. Choose the answer that *best* applies. If no answer is the perfect fit, pick whichever is the closest.

1. **When you read a business or personal development book and find it valuable, how often do you implement at least one of the strategies you've read?**

   (A) Always or almost always (at least 75% of the time).

   (B) Around 50% to 75%.

(C) My self-help book collection is mainly decorative. Less than 50% of the time.

(D) I don't read business or personal development books (or blogs).

2. **The last time you tried something new, how long had you been thinking about trying it before you did?**

(A) Less than a few weeks. I thought about it long enough to make sure the idea made sense but didn't delay taking action beyond that point.

(B) Between a few weeks and a few months.

(C) More than a few months.

(D) I don't pause before taking action. I'm a leap before I look type of person.

3. **When an appealing opportunity presents itself, what do you typically do?**

(A) Think, "I have similar skills to others who are already succeeding in the field, which is a great sign I can succeed at it too."

(B) A mixture of A and C.

(C) Create artificial roadblocks to acting. For example, I mind-read, thinking, "They probably have someone else in mind," without knowing if that's the case.

(D) I already told you, I'm a leap before I look type of person.

4. What's your ratio of successes to failures?

    (A) 50% to 70% of things I try are successes.

    (B) 71% to 99% of things I try are successes.

    (C) 100% of things I try are successes.

    (D) Less than 50% of things I try are successes.

5. When you think about things you've tried that haven't worked out, how do you feel?

    (A) I feel OK. I'm focused on achieving eventual mastery in important domains rather than perfect performance at all times. When I'm failing, I'm learning. My self-esteem can take the blow.

    (B) I feel embarrassed and bothered by thoughts about why I wasn't able to perform as well as I wanted to.

    (C) I doubt my capacity to ever be successful.

    (D) I blame it on other people.

6. Of the following six things, how many do you do?

- I have a tendency to procrastinate, even related to activities I enjoy.
- I avoid certain important activities.
- I recheck things excessively.
- I drive people nuts by frequently seeking reassurance.

- I partially commit to trying things.
- I seek information endlessly.

(A) None.

(B) One to two.

(C) Three to six.

(D) I'm the opposite of the person described.

Here's how to interpret your scores. If you scored:

Mostly A's

You're willing to act on ideas without long periods of hesitation. You have a moderate proportion of failures, indicating you're willing to learn through doing, which is one of the best and fastest ways to learn. You'll probably breeze through this chapter quickly.

Mostly B's

You're not permanently stuck on pause, but you tend to hesitate longer than is ideal. You may have more capacity for success than you realize, if you can train yourself to act on your good ideas sooner. The strategies in this chapter will help you recognize when you can act more swiftly than you usually would, without any major downsides to doing so. You're particularly likely to benefit from better understanding your thought processes around action taking and decision making, which this chapter will help you do.

Mostly C's

If you scored mostly C's, this chapter is ideally aimed at you. You fear failure. You probably have a feature of anxiety called *intolerance of uncertainty*, whereby you tend to avoid taking action until you feel 100% certain of what the path to success is.[1] You may find yourself perpetually stuck in the research phase of projects. You may contemplate many ideas without trying any of them, because you don't feel certain enough to commit to one idea. Try the suggestions in this chapter for ways to move your answers from C's to A's.

Mostly D's

Pausing too long before acting is unlikely to be one of your issues. In fact, you may have a tendency to under-reflect before taking action. This chapter will be less relevant to you than some of the other chapters, but because anxiety and impulsivity aren't mutually exclusive, you may still find it useful to read this chapter. That way, you'll pick up on the core anxiety concepts discussed here, which we'll build on in later chapters.

Being thoughtful, cautious, and introspective all have their advantages; however, sometimes there are benefits to being a hare instead of a tortoise. This chapter will help you understand the psychological mechanisms of why anxiety and hesitancy often go hand in hand. These mechanisms include overestimating the chances your actions will result in negative outcomes, catastrophizing failure, and becoming frozen or running away from situations in which you feel a sense of uncertainty.

. . . .

Thinking Shifts to Overcome Excessive Hesitancy

In this section, you'll do thought experiments that will make your thinking more balanced and flexible. These will help you feel motivated to take on the behavioral shifts, which follow later in the chapter. And remember: You don't need to do all of the experiments, just the ones that interest you.

Entertain the Idea That Your Actions Might Have Positive Consequences

You're thinking about painting your walls a color that's not white or cream. Your anxious mind is jumping to the negative prediction that you'll probably hate it and beat yourself up for having wasted the time and money. An alternative is that you'll love it, or at least quite like it, and it'll give you the confidence to try new ideas.

The tendency to predict that your actions will have negative outcomes is incredibly central to anxiety problems. If you can catch yourself when you're making a negative prediction and entertain alternatives, you'll likely ease a great deal of your anxiety. While there is a lot of information in this book, mastering this *one* simple principle will take you a very long way toward solving your anxiety issues. Pay close attention to this concept.

Whenever you're feeling anxious, use this feeling as your cue to practice articulating your negative prediction and an alternative. Try prompting yourself to think of the *best* possible outcome, instead of just the worst. You don't need to completely eliminate your fear; you just need to consider the different possibilities side by side, in an evenhanded way.

Experiment: For an action you'd like to take, try articulating both your feared negative outcome and an alternative possible outcome, just like the painting-the-walls example. If you practice this skill a lot, it will start to become a habit.

Feared outcome = _____

_____

Alternative outcome = _____

_____

Important: When you're attempting to shift your thoughts, picking a new thought that you want to strengthen is essential. Think of changing a thought as like attempting to change a habit: When you change a habit, you don't so much break a bad habit as build up and strengthen a new one.[2] When you practice entertaining new thoughts, eventually those new thoughts will start to become more automatic. In situations that used to trigger your old thoughts, now the new thought will also be triggered.

Recognize the Value of Acting *with* Uncertainty

Anxiety and uncertainty don't always mean you should stay stuck on pause. If you're currently stuck in pause mode, and have been for a while, taking some action is usually better than taking no action. When you can recognize the value of acting with uncertainty, you'll help your brain start to interpret uncertainty as a positive or not-so-terrible state, rather than it causing your alarm bells to ring loudly. The following is a thought experiment that's aimed at helping you recognize the value of acting even when you don't feel 100% sure of what the outcome will be or the exact best way to proceed.

Experiment: What are some circumstances in which acting with less than 100% certainty of success might be the best option? For example, submitting an application for a grant that will take four hours to prepare. You estimate the likelihood of obtaining the grant is only 10%, but it will be worth $5,000 if you're successful. Or trying a $50-a-month service that multiple people you trust have recommended. Or spending $100 on paint and painting supplies to see if you like a new room color. You've been thinking for years that you want to break out of off-white. Try to come up with three examples of your own. If coming up with three examples is intimidating, come up with just one example. Remember: You can adapt these instructions to suit yourself.

Recognize the Harm of Not Acting

People who are intolerant of uncertainty tend to work very hard to avoid harm. In other words, they'll jump through more hoops to avoid losing a dollar than to gain a dollar. You can work with your natural motivation if you begin to more carefully consider the harm of not acting. Naturally you may think of all the potential losses, costs, and risks of acting, but what about the costs, risks, and potential losses of *not* acting? Use the following question prompts to tune your attention to the costs of hesitation.

Experiment: These questions focus on what being hesitant has cost you in the past. I've written sample answers to help stimulate your thoughts. Try writing your own examples, one per question. The more specific and concrete your examples are the better. Don't be too hard on yourself about past mistakes.

Question	Sample Answers
1. What has hesitating cost you in terms of your time and mental energy?	You estimate you've been spending about four hours a week thinking about decisions you could've made already. [I like to assign a number or estimated number to each example, when applicable, to make the example more specific and objective.]
2. How would you have preferred to spend the time and/or energy you identified in question 1?	Getting more sleep, relaxing on the sofa more, watching more TV. [Hey, whatever floats your boat.]

Question	Sample Answers
3. What are the opportunities you've missed out on in the past due to hesitating?	Two years ago you considered buying a house down the road as an investment property. In the end, you couldn't push the button on the decision. The house has increased $50,000 in value in that time. [See how I again added the number to make the point more specific and objective.]
4. Has delaying or avoiding action had any interpersonal costs for you?	• Your friends get frustrated with you because you talk about ordering something different at your usual restaurants, but then always order the same dishes. • Your relationship partner also gets frustrated with you about your hesitancy in making decisions.
5. Have you found that the more you've avoided taking action, the less confident you've become? Have you developed more fear of failure? [*Hint:* One indicator that you've become more fearful of failure is if your perfectionism has increased over time.]	You remember you used to be more confident making friends than you are now.
6. What opportunities to learn from action have you lost while you've been stuck in nonaction mode?	You've delayed stock market investing. Now you're in your 40s and have a large sum to invest, but you have no experience in direct investing. You could've gained this experience by practicing when you had smaller amounts.

Question the Thought "Failure = Catastrophe"

Sometimes when you predict you'll experience a negative outcome, that prediction comes true. However, in reality, the vast majority of failures aren't catastrophes. When failure could result in a genuine catastrophe (for example, you're investing $100,000), that's a good reason to proceed very cautiously. However, you'll experience more success if you can distinguish between those situations and noncritical failures and mistakes.

Experiment: Think of something that your anxious mind is currently labeling as "would be a catastrophe." Possible examples include being told no, getting negative feedback, performing less than exceptionally well, or investing small amounts of money without getting a return. Where you're currently catastrophizing failure, try generating an alternative thought that you'd like to strengthen. For example:

OLD thought: "Attempting to do X and regretting it would be a disaster."

NEW thought: "Attempting to do X and regretting it would be upsetting, but tolerable."

Question the Thought "I Couldn't Cope with Trying Something and It Not Working Out"

This thinking shift is similar to but subtly different from the one just discussed. Many people underestimate their capacity to cope with trying something and not succeeding. Anxious people often worry about later regretting decisions and finding it hard to deal with the ensuing emotions. Solving this issue is often just a matter of realizing you could actually cope with mistakes, setbacks, and disappointments.

For example, you can see how good the human capacity is for coping with failure if you look at Olympians. *Advance warning:* I'm going to be a bit blunt here to make the point. Although only one person wins the gold medal in any Olympics event, the rest of the field don't go off and commit suicide or drink themselves into oblivion. Olympians are some of the most competitive, hard-driving people on the planet, and their personal investment is massive, yet they manage to cope and move on if their gold-medal dreams don't work out. It's not like all their training is wasted. The experiences and psychological skills (tenacity, precision, dedication, and so on) the person gains along the way means that it isn't.

Experiment: Think of past experiences when you successfully coped with emotions stemming from failures and mistakes—emotions like embarrassment, disappointment, sadness, and frustration. For example, someone broke up with you. At the time you couldn't imagine there would be a point when you would be over it, but now you are.

Tip: If you get stuck thinking about how you coped badly initially, ask yourself what you did after that. How did you pull yourself out of it eventually? Sometimes the answer is just that you got on with things and time passed.

On a positive note, if you can clearly see that you could cope with trying something and it not working out as you'd hoped, that's very empowering for making the decision to try it.

Question the Thought
"Failure = Never Going to Succeed"

Anxiety tends to make people think in dichotomous, either/or terms. A common example is seeing success and failure as the only two potential end points, rather than seeing a zigzagging path toward success that is dotted with failures along the way. Overcoming excessive hesitancy means learning to see failure as part of the path to eventual success.

To develop more tolerance of failure, you'll need what's called a *growth mindset*. A growth mindset means you believe you can improve your capabilities through the right kinds of practice. The alternative to a growth mindset is termed a *fixed mindset*. If you have a fixed mindset, you believe your capacities are fixed. People who have fixed mindsets are excessively scared of failure because they believe they can't improve. There's lots of research showing that people who have a growth mindset achieve more than people who have a fixed mindset.[3] The good news: People can successfully shift from fixed to growth mindsets.

Experiment: Try the following thought exercises to start shifting toward a growth mindset.

1. Have you had any past experiences where you ended up succeeding after initial failure? List one.

2. Identify one area in which you have a fixed mindset. It should be a skill/capacity you see as important to your success, where you see yourself as not as good as you'd like to be, and where you see that skill/capacity as fixed.

3. Identify a new growth mindset that you'd like to strengthen. For example, your old fixed mindset might be "I'm no good at negotiating." Your new mindset might be "I can improve at negotiating through practicing in a way that's a good fit with my temperament and values."

OLD thought: _____

_____

NEW thought: _____

_____

Question the Thought "Failure Is Just for Losers"

A failure-related thinking error that anxious perfectionists sometimes make is thinking that failure is just for losers. If you have this thinking bias, try this thought experiment:

Experiment: Think of a highly successful person you admire. It can be anyone, from Oprah to someone you actually know.

What failures has this person experienced in areas where he or she is generally successful? Has a businessperson you admire made some bad investments? Has your favorite actor made a movie that lost money? Has your favorite musician had an album flop?

You may be able to think of examples of failures off the top of your head, or you may need to do some online research or read a biography of that person. Make sure the examples are relevant to the person's core domain of success. A superstar chef opening a restaurant and failing is more relevant than an actor opening a restaurant and failing.

After you've done the thought experiment, ask yourself, "What's an alternative thought that's more realistic and less harsh than 'Failure is just for losers'?"

Alternate option: Ask mentors (people you actually know) about examples of their failures. Ask them what they learned from the experiences. You could also ask your mentors for examples of failures that have happened to prominent people in your field. They might be more willing to volunteer this information than to talk about their own failures.

Trust Your Gut

Gut instincts provide valuable information about when to say go and when to say no. However, "trust your gut" can be a very confusing message for anxiety-prone people because they find it hard to distinguish between gut instincts and anxiety symptoms. If you learn to recognize what your common anxiety patterns are when it comes to making decisions, you can distinguish these from your other gut instincts.

For example, let's say that whenever you're about to book an international flight you feel physically sick, but you always feel better as soon as you've pushed the "confirm purchase" button. If you can identify this sequence of emotions as a recurring pattern, you can recognize that your physical anxiety symptoms in these situations are usually a false alarm and not likely to mean that something is really wrong.

When you're in this type of situation, what gut instincts can you tune into that will tell you the decision to act is a good idea? What does a gut feeling to push "go" or say "yes" feel like to you? For me, a "go" instinct usually feels sort of tingly and excited, combined with some anxiety sensations (which are virtually always there when I'm making a decision to do something new). Pay attention to what your gut instinct to say yes feels like in your mind and body.

Of course, you also need to pay attention to when your gut instincts are giving you a valid "stop, something's wrong" message. A gut instinct in favor of stopping what you're currently doing might be a sense that until now you've been following a conventional path but one that isn't consistent with your passions or core strengths. A gut instinct that something is wrong might be a sense that something you're being told doesn't add up to you. Don't bury your instinct to seek clarification.

When you start paying attention, you'll notice that these other gut instincts feel different from your frozen-by-fear and analysis-paralysis feelings. These other instincts will clue you in about which action you should take.

Experiment: As you move through this book, start to identify how your general anxiety patterns differ from gut instincts that are likely to indicate something valid about the specific situation.

. . . .

Behavioral Shifts to Overcome Excessive Hesitancy

Important: So far we've been focusing on how tweaking your thinking can help shift your behavior. This is important, but it's only half the story. People are usually quite good at identifying how changes in thoughts or feelings may lead to changes in behavior, such as "When I have more energy, I'll do more exercise" or "When I have more ideas, I'll take more action." However, people tend to underestimate the impact of changing their behavior on their thoughts and feelings, such as "When I exercise more, I'll have more energy" or "When I take more action, I'll have more ideas." Don't make the mistake of thinking you need to wait for your thoughts to change before you try behavioral shifts. Mental and behavioral shifts go hand in hand. When you start making changes in your behavior (even subtle ones), you'll notice that all kinds of thoughts, including your view of yourself, start to shift. Changing your behavior, without waiting for your thoughts to always shift first, is one of the best and fastest ways you can reduce your anxiety. That's why a cognitive behavioral approach focuses on both thoughts and behaviors.

The behavioral changes we're going to discuss in this section will help you develop a better balance between acting and thinking, but first let's look at a strategy you can use to decrease anxious feelings, no matter what their cause.

Decrease Anxiety in an Instant

The best way to instantly feel less anxious is to slow your breathing. Try this whenever you feel physically overaroused due to anxiety, or when your thoughts are either racing or frozen. Slowing your breathing will automatically slow down your heart rate. You'll feel calmer. Since this is a physiological fact, it's about the only anxiety strategy that has a 100% guarantee of working. The effect is nearly instant.

Here are some tips for slowing your breathing:

1. Before you try to slow your breathing, drop your shoulders. It'll make it easier. Also, focus on breathing slowly rather than breathing deeply.

2. If you have an area of tension in your body, like your neck and shoulders are tight, imagine you're breathing fresh new air into those areas. There's nothing sciencey about this, but lots of people like this method.

3. My favorite way to show people that slow breathing is working is to use a free smartphone app to measure their heart rate (see TheAnxietyToolkit.com/resources). The app works by sticking your finger over the camera lens on your phone. The camera picks up your pulse by detecting tiny changes

in blood flow in your finger. You can view your heart rate on your phone and see if it's trending down. Be aware that your heart rate is naturally slightly faster when you're breathing in, compared to when you're breathing out.

Decide When and Where You'll Act

Since anxious people usually assume the worst, they tend to assume changes can be achieved only through enormous amounts of effort. However, psychology research is full of examples of how huge improvements can be achieved through tiny shifts made at key decision points. Here's one example of this:

Deciding when and where you're going to do something will dramatically increase the likelihood you'll follow through. Let's look at the results from a specific study.[4] Because most psychology research uses students as guinea pigs, this example relates to essay writing. Students who had an essay to complete were divided into two groups. One group was asked to state when and where they would complete their essay. Of this group, 71% completed the essay before the due date. The other group was given the due date but were not asked to state when and where they'd write their essay. Only 32% of this group finished on time. This extremely simple, two-minute intervention transformed the task from one in which most people failed to one in which most people succeeded.

To implement this change in your own life, whenever you're planning to take action, identify when and where you'll act. Make this a habit you do every time.

Expose Yourself to Success Experiences

Consider this: A child asks her mom for a bag of M&M's at the supermarket. If her mom even occasionally says yes, the child will be motivated to try the request again in the future. This pattern is called *intermittent reinforcement*. Intermittent reinforcement means sometimes getting rewarded but without being able to predict when you'll score vs. when you'll strike out.[5]

Intermittent reinforcement results in behaviors being quickly acquired and creates behaviors that are very persistent—just ask a mom who has caved in to candy requests a few times. You can also see the intermittent reinforcement principle in people who buy lottery tickets and who experience the occasional win. Their wins provide a jolt of dopamine, fix their attention toward the potential for winning big, and reinforce their continued "effort" of buying tickets.

The take-home message: Even if you achieve only intermittent reinforcement—that is, you experience success only sometimes—having some successes will make your behavior much more resilient, and you'll be less likely to give up. Therefore, whenever you start something, focus on getting your first few successes. For example, if you desire success in the business domain, focus on getting your first few clients, your first few sales, or your first few experiences of getting a pitch accepted. Focus on these things ahead of perfecting your pricing structure, your website, your media kit, and so on. Give yourself a taste of success.

Surround Yourself with Others Who Are Already Doing What You Want to Do

My all-time favorite success tip for people who tend to hesitate excessively is to regularly interact with people who are already successfully doing what you want to do. Why will this help you moderate your tortoise tendencies? Emotions, thoughts, and behaviors all tend to be socially contagious.[6] Therefore, if you surround yourself with people who are already acting in the ways you need to act, this will likely rub off on you. You'll be more likely to take action.

Another key reason for interacting with others who are already succeeding in your field is that many of the key pieces of information that will help you succeed won't be shared in books or other public forums. They're likely passed from person to person. You'll get to know these insider secrets only by befriending successful people.

Practice Tolerating Uncertainty

Look for opportunities to try taking action when you're not 100% certain of success. Gradually experiment with this over the coming months as opportunities come up. The more you learn from experience that you're capable of doing this, the easier it will become. Taking action swiftly will start to feel more natural. When an opportunity to act with uncertainty comes up, articulate the potential upsides of taking action:

- It could work out well.
- If it doesn't work out well, I'll move my thinking forward by seeing that the idea didn't work.
- I won't have to think about the decision anymore.

Practice Hesitating Less

Look for small ways to practice hesitating a little less than you usually would. Over time, this will help increase your psychological flexibility: You'll get better at choosing when you want to let a decision marinate vs. when you want to make a decision swiftly, take action, and move on. You'll start to learn from experience that you can move out of thinking mode more quickly without disastrous consequences. For example, if you tend to put off buying things that, in reality, would be a good investment, give yourself some criteria for making quicker decisions. You might commit to making decisions about purchases that are under $50 in less than 48 hours. Choose the level that suits your situation and preferences.

CHAPTER 5

Rumination

How to Get Your Thinking Unstuck

Anxiety often leads to two types of overthinking: rumination (mentally replaying events that have happened, in either the recent or the distant past) and worry (fear about what may happen in the future). This chapter will help you learn to cope effectively whenever you get caught in these anxiety traps.

Take the following quiz to see how this chapter pertains to you. Choose the answer that *best* applies. If no answer is the perfect fit, pick whichever is the closest.

1. **How often do you find yourself mentally replaying conversations from the *recent* past (including email, texting, and IMing)?**

   (A) Never or rarely.

   (B) Sometimes, but less than once a week.

   (C) At least weekly.

2. **How often do you find yourself mentally replaying negative events that happened in the *nonrecent* past (things that happened months or years ago)?**

   (A) Never or rarely.

   (B) Sometimes, but less than once a fortnight.

   (C) At least once a fortnight.

3. **Do you ever feel physically sick with anxiety?**

   (A) No, or extremely rarely.

   (B) During transition points in my life (for example, starting a new job) but not generally.

   (C) Once a month or more.

4. **What do you do after a high-stakes performance situation (such as giving an important talk, audition, or interview) that didn't go as well as you'd hoped?**

   (A) Plan how I'll implement simple changes for next time.

   (B) Have a glass of wine and attempt to forget about it.

   (C) Spend weeks obsessing over what I could've done better and worrying about how I was perceived.

5. **When you think about your weaknesses, how do you react?**

   (A) Recognize that weaknesses are part of the universal human experience.

(B) Hope no one will notice my flaws.

(C) Spend hours worrying that my weaknesses will prevent me from having the success and happiness I desire.

6. **What do you do when you realize you've made a significant error?**

(A) Fix it and move on.

(B) Put corrective action in place but lose some nights' sleep over it.

(C) Stress about it, but I'm so frozen by anxiety I often don't put corrective action in place.

Here's how to interpret your scores. If you scored:

Mostly A's

Rumination isn't a major problem for you. When you can see ways you can improve, you make specific plans about when and where you're going to implement your brain waves. You can probably move through this chapter quickly; however, there should be at least a few nuggets of insight you can take away.

Mostly B's

Rumination is an occasional problem for you. Learning strategies for coping when upsetting things happen will help you feel more relaxed. Although rumination and worry aren't all-consuming aspects of your life, they're not pleasant states, and there are some easy techniques you can learn and keep in your toolkit for when you need them.

Mostly C's

You're regularly sucked into the rumination vortex. You reflect a lot about ways you could be more successful, but you don't tend to plan how you'll implement those ideas. Rumination and worry get in the way of useful idea generation and problem solving. The strategies in this chapter will help you make large reductions in the amount of time you spend ruminating and worrying, and will help you make more effective choices.

Believe it or not, psychologists have a term to describe people who like to think a lot. The trait is called *need for cognition*. It refers to people who enjoy effortful thinking and feel motivated to attempt to understand and make sense of things. Because you're reading a book about understanding yourself and your thoughts, chances are you fall into this category.

For the most part, being high in need for cognition is associated with positive traits, like openness, higher self-esteem, and lower social anxiety.[1] On the flipside, some other types of intensive thinking—notably rumination and worry—tend to be associated with being closed to new ideas and poor mental health. This chapter aims to help you with unhelpful overthinking. The intention is for you to be able to enjoy and benefit from useful self-reflection and other types of deep thinking, without getting tangled in knots of worry and self-criticism.

. . . .

Thinking Shifts to Navigate Rumination and Worry

Anxiety and rumination form a feedback loop where one causes the other. Here you'll learn to recognize when you're ruminating so you can disrupt the loop. We'll also cover some very simple mindfulness exercises you can use to develop a more nonstick mind.

Identify When You're Ruminating

To reduce your rumination, you're first going to need to identify it. Rumination can be about minor issues:

Why did I pay $4.20 for gas at the first gas station off the highway when I could've driven a half mile down the road and paid $3.60? I shouldn't have been so stupid. I should've realized that the gas station closest to the freeway exit would be more expensive than the others in town. Why did I let myself get sucked in by the fact that so many other people were fueling up there? Why were so many other people prepared to pay such excessive prices anyway? Are we all just sheep?

Rumination can also be more heavy-duty self-criticism:

What's wrong with me? I have these dreams, but I don't make them happen. Am I just full of hot air? Maybe I don't want them bad enough? Am I just a big fraud?

Ruminating can sometimes be a bit like daydreaming, in that people often get lost in rumination without realizing they're doing it. Try the next experiment to improve your ability to detect rumination.

Experiment: Jot down a list of the different topics of rumination you're prone to. Use the following ideas to brainstorm, or just fill in the blanks:

- Replaying conversations with people in power positions in your life. For example, replaying conversations, including email conversations, with [insert names of people] _____.
- Replaying memories of experiences of failure from the past. For example, _____.
- Thinking about ways in which you're not as perfect as you'd like to be. For example, thinking you're not as good at _____ as you'd like.
- Thinking about things you should be doing to be more successful, such as _____.
- Thinking about whether you're too much of a loser to ever have success and happiness.
- Replaying small errors you've made, such as _____.
- Thinking about the path not taken, such as _____.

If you think of more types or examples, you can add them later. The goal of this initial exercise isn't to change your rumination; it's only to help you know what you're trying to spot.

Become Aware of Memory Bias

When people are anxious, they often have biased recall for events.[2] For example, Brian talks himself into believing he screwed up an interview for a promotion because he thinks over and over about things he could've said. However, he doesn't as easily recall the good answers he gave. He endlessly mentally rehashes ambiguous cues the interviewers gave off, such as appearing to rush through questions, but doesn't as easily recall when the interviewers responded positively.

Another example: A friend of mine used to talk herself into believing she'd failed every exam she ever took. She'd ruminate over all the answers she hadn't known and wouldn't recall questions she'd been able to answer correctly. The take-home message when you're ruminating: Don't trust your memory. You might be ruminating about something fictional or at least magnified. This also applies to ruminating about how you think others perceive you; you may just be mind reading based on a biased memory of interactions.

Experiment: Do you have any current rumination topics where memory bias might be playing a role? If you can't think of anything now, come back to this experiment when you have an issue that fits. Answer the following questions:

1. What's your ruminating mind telling you?

2. What are the objective data telling you about whether your ruminative thoughts are likely to be correct? For example, my friend who always convinced herself she'd failed exams had never failed anything.

3. Are you recalling feedback as harsher than it was or recalling blips in your performance as worse than they were?

Distinguish Between Worry/Rumination and Helpful Problem Solving

If you're smart and you've experienced a lifetime of being rewarded for your thinking skills, it makes sense that you'll default to trying to think your way out of emotional pain. However, because anxiety tends to make thinking negative, narrow, and rigid, it's difficult to do creative problem solving when you're feeling highly anxious. People who are heavy worriers tend to believe that worrying helps them make good decisions.[3] However, rather than helping you problem-solve, rumination and worry usually just make it difficult to see the forest for the trees.

Do you think people who worry a lot about getting cancer are more likely to do self-exams, have their moles mapped, or eat a healthy diet? According to research, the opposite is probably true. Worriers and ruminators wait longer before taking action. For example, one study showed that women who were prone to rumination took an average of 39 days longer to seek help after noticing a breast lump.[4] That's a scary thought.

If you think about it, worry often comes from lack of confidence in being able to handle situations. Here's an example: Technophobes who worry a lot about their hard drives crashing are the same people who are scared of accidentally wiping all their files if they attempt to do a backup. Therefore, worry is often associated with *not* doing effective problem solving. My experience of dealing with technophobic ruminators is that they don't usually back up their computers!

Experiment: To check for yourself whether ruminating and worrying lead to useful actions, try tracking the time you spend ruminating or worrying for a week. If a week is too much of a commitment, you could try two days—one weekday and one weekend day. When you notice yourself ruminating or worrying, write down the approximate number of minutes you spend doing it. The following day, note any times when ruminating/worrying led to useful solutions. Calculate your ratio: How many minutes did you spend overthinking for each useful solution it generated?

Reduce Self-Criticism

Reducing self-criticism is a critical part of reducing rumination. Self-criticism is a fuel source for your rumination fire. People use self-criticism to try to encourage themselves to do better in the future. For example, someone might ruminate after overeating or if she perceives she has mucked up a social situation, and then mentally beat herself up about her mistakes. However, harsh self-criticism doesn't help you move forward because it isn't a very effective motivational tool, especially if you're already ruminating.[5]

People who are in a pattern of trying to use self-criticism as motivation often fear that reducing it will make them lazy. It won't. In fact, giving yourself a compassionate rather than a critical message will often lead to working harder. For example, one study showed that people who took a hard test and got a compassionate message afterward were willing to study longer for a future similar test, compared to a group of people who took the same test but didn't get a compassionate message.[6]

Giving yourself a simple "don't be too hard on yourself" message will propel you toward taking useful problem-solving steps. Acknowledging the emotions you're feeling (such as embarrassed, disappointed, upset) and then giving yourself compassion will lead to your making better choices than criticizing yourself will. Self-compassion will give you the clear mental space you need to make good decisions.

Experiment: To practice using self-compassion as an alternative to self-criticism, try the following three-minute writing exercise.

There are two versions of this exercise—one that involves thinking about a past mistake and another that involves thinking about something you perceive as a major weakness. Identify a mistake or weakness that you want to focus on, and then write for three minutes using the following instructions: "Imagine that you are talking to yourself about this weakness (or mistake) from a compassionate and understanding perspective. What would you say?"

Try this experiment now, or store it away for a future situation in which you find yourself ruminating about a mistake or weakness. This experiment comes from the same series of research studies as the one involving the hard test mentioned earlier. Note that the study participants didn't receive training in how to write compassionate messages. What they naturally came up with in response to the prompt worked.

Recognize When You're Criticizing Yourself Just for Feeling Anxious

Should/shouldn't thinking traps are a common problem for anxiety-prone people. These can come in several varieties, virtually all of which can prolong and intensify rumination—for example, "I shouldn't ever let anyone down," which is an example of excessive responsibility taking and rigid thinking.

Try to notice when you get caught in should/shouldn't thinking traps, in which you criticize yourself just for feeling anxious. For example, "I should be able to handle life much better" or "I shouldn't get anxious about such little issues." If this happens, give yourself compassion for the fact that you feel anxious, regardless of whether the anxiety is logical or not. Think of it this way: If a kid was scared of monsters, you wouldn't withhold compassion and empathy just because the monsters aren't real. Treat yourself with the same caring. A common mistake people make is to think they need to give themselves excessive encouragement, praise, or pep talks while they're feeling anxious—you don't. Taking a patient and compassionate attitude about the fact that you're experiencing anxiety is an overlooked strategy that helps anxious feelings pass quickly.

Experiment: When you're ruminating, do you ever further dump on yourself by criticizing yourself for feeling anxious? Try this: Switch out any *shoulds* hidden in your self-talk and replace them with *prefer*.[7] For example, instead of saying "I should have achieved more by now" try "I would prefer to have achieved more by now."

This is a simple, specific, repeatable example of how you can talk to yourself in a kinder, more patient way. These tiny self-interventions may seem ridiculously simple, but they work. They may not seem like they shift your anxiety to a huge degree; however, they can help you disrupt your rumination just enough to give you a small window of clear mental space. This allows you to start doing something useful rather than keep ruminating. Doing something useful then further helps lift you out of rumination. You get a positive feedback loop (positive thoughts ➔ positive behavior ➔ positive thoughts) rather than a negative loop.

Spot Rumination Triggered by Emails

Email is a common trigger for rumination. Text messages, Facebook comments, and tweets can be too. All the nonverbal cues, and many of the context cues, are stripped out of this type of communication. The asynchronized nature of email often adds to the issue.

For example, does a slow reply to an email mean the person is disinterested? Or might it mean something else? Is the person busy? A habitual slow replier? Waiting on some information before coming back to you with a reply? Still thinking about what you've said? Is the person disorganized and got distracted? Not checking messages? Did your message go to spam?

If you get caught in email-induced rumination, recognize if you're jumping to any negative conclusions about why the person hasn't responded and try coming up with alternative explanations that are plausible. Use the next experiment as a guide. Remember that slowing your breathing will always help you think more clearly and flexibly, so do this too.

Experiment: Can you recall a time when a nontimely response to an email set off rumination for you? What was (1) your worst-case scenario prediction for the person's lack of response, (2) the best-case scenario, and (3) the most likely scenario?[8] If you struggle to think of an answer for "most likely," pick something that falls in the middle, between your answers for the best- and worst-case scenarios.

In the email incident you just recalled, did you ever find out what the reason for the slow response was? Often you won't find out the reasons for other people's actions, which is part of why this type of rumination tends to be so futile. More on this next.

Accept That You Often Won't Know Why Other People Have Acted in a Particular Way

Humans like to have explanations for why things happen. When we don't have one, we tend to invent something. Sometimes the explanations involve personalizing. *Personalizing* is when you take something more personally than it was meant in reality. If a work colleague is rude and abrupt, you might think it's because she's annoyed at you, and not consider that it might be because she's feeling flustered by something unrelated. Anxiety-prone people who don't like uncertainty can be especially likely to ruminate about why something has happened and come up with explanations involving excessive personalizing. To overcome this, you need to learn to tolerate that you're not always going to know why people behave the way they do.

Recognize that if someone acts strangely, there's a very high likelihood that the behavior has something to do with what's happening for that person, rather than being about you, and you're probably never going to know what the reason was. You can save yourself hours or days of rumination and upset if you can tolerate the idea of not knowing. While there might be some cases in which you try to find out what the issue was, in many cases your only real choice is to let it go. Try to arrive at this insight before you've done hours of ruminating!

Experiment: Was there a time recently when in retrospect it would've been better to accept not knowing the reason for someone's ambiguous behavior rather than trying to figure it out?

Try Mindfulness Meditation

Mindfulness meditation is like Tylenol, in that the same treatment is capable of helping with multiple issues: decreasing anxiety-induced overarousal, boosting your focus, and improving your ability to detect rumination. Mindfulness-based therapies have been shown to be effective for helping people reduce anxiety.[9]

Mindfulness meditation does not need to be intimidating. Research by the makers of the Lift goal-tracking app found that beginner meditators start with an average of three to five minutes.[10] They also found that once people had meditated 12 times, there was around a 90% chance they'd do more meditation.

Experiment: Explore and find a version of meditation that works for you. Start with three minutes of one of the following practices, and increase the time you spend meditating by 30 seconds each day:

- Pay attention to the physical sensations of your breathing. Lie down and put your hand on your abdomen to feel the sensations of it rising as you breathe in and falling as you breathe out.
- Sit or lie down and listen to any sounds and the silence between sounds. Let sounds just come in and out of your

awareness regardless of whether they're relaxing sounds
or not.

- Walk for three minutes and pay attention to what you see.
- Walk and pay attention to the feelings of air on your skin.
- Walk and pay attention to the physical sensations of your
  body moving.
- Do three minutes of open awareness, in which you pay
  attention to any sensations that show up. Pay attention
  to anything in the here and now, which could be sounds,
  your breathing, the sensations of your body making contact with your chair, or the sensations of your feet on the
  floor.
- Spend three minutes paying attention to any sensations of
  pain, tension, comfort, or relaxation in your body. You don't
  need to try to change the sensations; just allow them to be
  what they are, and ebb and flow as they do.

When your thoughts drift away from what you're supposed
to be paying attention to, gently (and without self-criticism) bring
them back. Expect to need to do this a lot. It's a normal part of
doing mindfulness meditation and doesn't mean you're doing it
wrong.

You're likely to get more benefits from meditation if you do
it on a regular basis and for longer amounts of time per session.
However, in all honesty, I mostly use it just when I feel busy,
antsy, and scattered, and need some help to calm my thoughts.
If you want to use meditation on an as-needed basis, try doing it
daily for 30 days so that you get the hang of it first. When you've

practiced meditation regularly for a period of time, it will come much more naturally when you want to use it.

If you attempt to meditate when you're already ruminating or when your thoughts are racing (for example, due to having too much to do), it may not feel very relaxing. However, it will still be working.

Define Your Options

When people are spinning their rumination wheels about a particular problem, they often don't concretely define what their options are for moving forward. To shift out of rumination and into problem-solving mode, concretely and realistically define what your best three to six options are. For example, imagine you've recently hired a new employee but that person is not working out. Instead of mentally slapping yourself around about why you made the hire, it would be more useful to define what your options are at this point:

- Giving the employee more time
- Shifting the employee's responsibilities to simpler jobs
- Giving the employee checklists of the steps needed to complete each task
- Having another employee work with the individual
- Firing the employee

Defining your options relieves some of the stress of rumination and helps you shift to effective problem solving. Keeping your list of options short will prevent you from running into choice-overload problems. Research shows that if you consider more than three to six choices, you're less likely to end up making a choice.[11]

Experiment: Practice concretely defining your best three to six options for moving forward with a problem you're currently ruminating or worrying about. Write brief bullet points, like in the example just given. You can use this method for all sorts of problems. For example, a friend just used it to come up with ideas for how to have more social contact in her life.

Note: If the word *best* is causing you to jump into perfectionism/frozen mode, write any three to six options.

Use Imagery Exposure If Ruminative Thoughts Have Become Very, Very Stuck

If past situations keep playing on your mind and other strategies aren't working for you, you can use a technique called *imagery exposure*. This is a clinical technique used in therapy, so in this instance, stick to the instructions rather than adapting them. Read through these instructions in full before deciding if you want to give this technique a try. It's heavy duty but often very effective.

Imagery exposure is a technique in which you vividly recall a situation you've been ruminating about, such as a colleague pointing out an embarrassing error you made. You can also use imagery exposure for a worry thought (something that hasn't happened yet).

To start, recall all the sights and sounds of the past situation (or feared situation) in as much detail as you can. For example, if you're recalling a situation that has happened, you might recall turning bright red with embarrassment and the other people looking at you strangely or laughing. You would also recall details like what the room looked like, what the temperature was, whether the sun was streaming in through the window, and so on. Bring the image of the embarrassing or worry situation vividly to mind.

The following is based on the principle that anxiety symptoms will naturally subside if you don't use escape or avoidance strategies: Deliberately keep the image in mind until your anxiety falls to half of where it started (or less). For example, if vividly recalling the situation triggers 8 out of 10 anxiety initially, hold the image in mind until your anxiety drops to about a level 4. Repeat the imagery exposure exercise at least once a day until you can bring the image to mind without it triggering more than about half of the peak anxiety you experienced the first time you tried imagery exposure.

Exposure techniques like this are some of the most powerful ways to solve problems with intrusive thoughts when an event is still bothering you long after it happened. Only use the technique if you feel like you can handle it. You can use imagery exposure for recent memories or more distant ones. If you have actual trauma to deal with, I hope you'll use common sense and have a therapist help you deal with those kinds of memories. Similar exposure-based procedures are effective for trauma memories, but a therapist who is experienced in treating trauma will help you monitor the intensity of the procedure so you don't become excessively overwhelmed during the process.

. . . .

Behavioral Shifts to Navigate Rumination and Worry

Take Action If You're Ruminating Because of Avoidance Coping

If you're ruminating because you've been putting off dealing with an issue, taking any level of action to address what you've been avoiding will usually help alleviate your rumination. Most of the time, you won't need to completely resolve the issue to lift your rumination—for example, you might just send an email or make a phone call to get the ball rolling. If your rumination is being triggered by avoidance coping, see Chapter 8 for more insights and strategies.

Replace Behaviors That Make Your Rumination and Worry Worse

There's not much point in using strategies to decrease rumination and worry if you're concurrently adding fuel to those fires. Self-criticism is one kind of fuel. Other types of fuel include things like excessive reassurance seeking, spending hours looking up health information online, or compulsively looking at your ex's Facebook page.

Look out for behaviors that seem to provide a temporary reprieve from anxiety but, in fact, make you feel like you need to go back and repeat them. Look into seeing a cognitive behavioral therapist if you can't stop these behaviors on your own.

Reduce Overthinking by Capturing Ideas as You Have Them

If you have a smartphone, use a note-taking app to capture ideas as you have them. Doing this relieves the stress of trying to remember them later. It prevents the frustration of remembering you had a great thought but not being able to recall what it was, and it frees up your mental work pad for more ideas.

Like any anti-anxiety strategy, you can overdo note taking. If you find that your note taking becomes obsessive, you feel anxious when you can't write something down, or you end up with lists that are so long that processing them becomes stressful and you can't address the issue on your own, consider seeking professional guidance.

Move Ruminative Thinking Forward by Asking Questions

Have you ever had the experience of asking someone for advice and then realizing you could've figured out a solution yourself? You can use this effect to your advantage. Ask questions as a way of unclogging stuck thinking. When you ask questions, you may get useful new information, or just the process of asking the questions may stimulate your own thinking.

Sometimes even getting unhelpful responses can help you move forward, because they prompt you to define your problem differently. This often happens when someone misunderstands your question and gives an unhelpful, irrelevant response, but this makes you reformulate your question in a clearer form.

Ways you can ask questions include making phone calls, scheduling an appointment with an adviser, posting your questions on Facebook or an online forum, or hiring someone you can direct questions to. For example, when my brother-in-law was teaching himself computer programming, he hired a more experienced programmer he could ask questions of whenever he got stuck. It was a brilliant strategy and much cheaper than taking a college course!

CHAPTER 6

· ·

Paralyzing Perfectionism

How to Stop Getting Derailed by the Wrong Kinds of High Standards

When you're working hard on achieving your goals, the ideal scenario is that you enjoy the successes you experience along the way and take setbacks in stride. However, anxiety-related perfectionism can get in the way. This chapter will help you learn to focus on the big picture. You'll learn alternative coping strategies to prevent you from getting caught up in unhelpful types of perfectionism.

Take the following quiz to see how this chapter pertains to you. Choose the answer that *best* applies. If no answer is the perfect fit, pick whichever is the closest.

1. How often are you bothered by fears of not being good enough?

(A) Never.

(B) Sometimes.

(C) Often.

2. **How often are you bothered by things that aren't important in the big scheme of things?**

   (A) Never.

   (B) Sometimes.

   (C) Often.

3. **How often do you become frustrated with the pace of your success?**

   (A) Never or rarely.

   (B) Sometimes.

   (C) Often.

4. **What's your reaction when other people perform better than you?**

   (A) I might strive for outstanding performance, but I don't panic if other people perform better than I do some of the time.

   (B) When my peers have successes, it triggers some degree of social comparison anxiety for me.

   (C) If I don't perform better than everyone else, I tend to feel like a failure.

5. **When you're working on a large-scale, multiweek project and you start thinking, "I'm not sure if I can do this," what's your typical response?**

(A) I take a break and then identify some easy aspects of the task that I can tick off to get my confidence back.

(B) I worry that my negative thought might be true, but I keep working.

(C) I feel depressed, automatically jump to the conclusion that my pessimistic thought must be true, and spend the next hour browsing gossip sites on the Internet to soothe myself.

6. How successful are you at managing your willpower?

(A) I always keep some willpower available in my tank so I can keep my cool when dealing with unexpected situations.

(B) I don't lose it with other people, but I often feel like my willpower tank is on empty.

(C) I frequently run out of willpower and end up doing things I regret, often involving a pint of ice cream or yelling at loved ones.

7. Do you jump from unfinished project to unfinished project when self-doubt creeps in?

(A) No. I'm willing to quit a project, but based on objective data that it was a bad idea rather than self-doubt.

(B) Sometimes.

(C) Yes. My home and my hard drive are full of things I started and didn't finish.

———

Here's how to interpret your scores. If you scored:

Mostly A's

Perfectionism isn't a biggie for you. You seem to be good at managing your willpower and priorities and taking temporary setbacks in stride. You're confident about taking on any project that interests you. When self-doubt raises its head, you're able to see it as temporary. You'll probably fly through this chapter, but you're still likely to learn some interesting tidbits that will help you optimize your coping.

Mostly B's

There's room for improvement in how you manage your willpower, creativity, confidence, and energy. Most of the time, you're confident in your abilities, but when peers are experiencing success or you're frustrated with how something is progressing, it can trigger a degree of self-doubt and ineffective coping responses. The strategies in this chapter will help you keep your focus on the big picture, without getting thrown off course by setbacks and minor issues.

Mostly C's

Based on your answers, you struggle to manage your confidence and willpower when it comes to prioritizing work and coping with setbacks and imperfections. Self-doubt thoughts have a tendency to derail you, causing you to quit or overwork in ineffective ways. You feel confident only when you're outperforming your peers. The strategies in this chapter will help you move your answers from C's to A's.

Perfectionism is considered a risk factor for developing anxiety problems.[1] Not every anxious person is a perfectionist, but if you are, this chapter is for you.

. . . .

Thinking Shifts to Overcome Unhelpful Types of Perfectionism

Anxiety-related thinking patterns can contribute to problems like prioritizing the wrong types of tasks, feeling burned out, and getting intensely frustrated when results aren't coming as quickly or consistently as you'd like. I'll explain how below.

Catch Either/Or Thinking

Anxious perfectionists will typically think "I need to perform flawlessly at all times," with their underlying assumption being "or else it will result in disaster." This is a common type of thinking trap termed either/or thinking. In this case, the either/or is this: Either there is flawless performance or complete and utter failure, and nothing in between.

Not only can this style of thinking make you feel crushed

when you don't meet your own ideal standards, but it also often leads to perfectionism paralysis. Take, for example, an artist who sees his future career prospects as becoming either the next Picasso or a penniless flop; this person doesn't see other possible outcomes in between. You can see how this would give the artist a creative block.

For other folks, their hidden assumption may be slightly different: "Either I need to perform flawlessly at all times, or other people will reject me." When I look back at my clinical psychology training, I realize I had this belief at that time. At a semiconscious level, I thought that the only way to prevent getting booted out of the program was to score at the top of the class for every test or assignment.

Ultra-high standards often arise because a person is trying to hide imagined catastrophic flaws.[2] In this scenario, people often think that if their flaws get revealed they'll be shunned, and so the only way to conceal their defects is by always excelling. When people who have this belief do excel, their brain jumps to the conclusion that excelling was the only reason they managed to avoid catastrophe. This then perpetuates their belief that excelling is necessary for preventing future disasters.

Researchers have used the term *clinical perfectionism* to describe the most problematic kind of perfectionism. When clinical perfectionists manage to meet their ultra-high standards, they often conclude that those standards must not have been high enough and revise them upward, meaning they can never feel any sense of peace.[3]

All this being said, I'm not suggesting you shoot for "acceptable" performance standards if you're capable of excellence. Most of the anxious perfectionists I've worked with would hate that. It's not in their nature to feel comfortable with mediocre performance. What I'm going to recommend in this chapter are some subtle tweaks to the types of standards you set for yourself. These tweaks will help you set standards that are equally ambitious (if not more so), but will prevent some of the problems caused by perfectionism.

Experiment: Ask yourself if the either/or perfectionism trap is a problem for you. If it is, consider the following:

1. Maybe the flaws you see yourself as having aren't as big in reality as they are in your mind. Maybe other people will care less about them than you think. Can you think of any flaws you perceive yourself as having where this might be true?

2. Achieving excellent performance at all times isn't a realistic option, nor is always performing at the top, especially if you're mixing in a pool of other smart people. Sometimes anxious perfectionists will avoid mixing with other very talented people because it triggers social comparison and self-doubt. This has a self-sabotaging effect because smart people spark each other's ideas (the iron sharpens iron principle). Do you avoid situations that trigger social comparison?

3. Give other people some credit. Why would they forget about all the other stellar work you've done if you

occasionally produce something that is not quite at your usual high standard?

Switch from a Performance Focus to a Mastery Focus

There's a way to keep your standards high but avoid the problems that come from perfectionism. If you can shift your thinking from a performance focus to a mastery focus, you'll become less fearful, more resilient, and more open to good, new ideas. *Performance focus* is when your highest priority is to show you can do something well now. *Mastery focus* is when you're mostly concerned with advancing your skills.[4] Someone with a mastery focus will think, "My goal is to master this skill set" rather than "I need to perform well to prove myself."

A mastery focus can help you persist after setbacks. To illustrate this, imagine the following scenario: Adam is trying to master the art of public speaking. Due to his mastery goal, he's likely to take as many opportunities as he can to practice giving speeches. When he has setbacks, he'll be motivated to try to understand these and get back on track. His mastery focus will make him more likely to work steadily toward his goal. Compare this with performance-focused Rob, who is concerned just with proving his competence each time he gives a talk. Rob will probably take fewer risks in his style of presentation and be less willing to step outside his comfort zone. If he has an incident in which a talk doesn't go as well as he'd hoped, he's likely to start avoiding public speaking opportunities.

Mastery goals will help you become less upset about individual instances of failure. They'll increase your willingness to identify where you've made errors, and they'll help you avoid becoming so excessively critical of yourself that you lose confidence in your ability to rectify your mistakes.

A mastery focus can also help you prioritize—you can say yes to things that move you toward your mastery goal and no to things that don't. This is great if you're intolerant of uncertainty, because it gives you a clear direction and rule of thumb for making decisions about which opportunities to pursue.

Experiment: What's your most important mastery goal right now? Complete this sentence: "My goal is to master the skills involved in _____." Examples include parenting, turning more website visitors into buyers, property investment, or self-compassion. Based on the mastery goal you picked, answer the following questions. Make your answers as specific as possible.

How would people with your mastery goal:

1. React to mistakes, setbacks, disappointments, and negative moods?

2. Prioritize which tasks they work on? What types of tasks would they deprioritize?

3. React when they'd sunk a lot of time into something and then realized a particular strategy or idea didn't have the potential they'd hoped it would?

4. Ensure they were optimizing their learning and skill acquisition?

5. React when they felt anxious?

Catch the Minimizing Thinking Error

Anxious perfectionists are prone to minimizing their achievements. For example, a chef might dismiss any awards short of a Michelin star as "not really that significant."

Experiment: Which of your achievements and skills do you tend to devalue? Could you feel more confident in yourself by viewing your existing achievements and skills more realistically, rather than minimizing them?

Accept the Pace of Success

Do you ever feel frustrated when you're not achieving success as quickly as you'd like? For example, after I graduated and moved to London, it took me a month to get a job. At the time, that seemed like forever. I was a walking ball of stress, counting every British pound I spent while I had no money coming in. Looking back, it seems nonsensical that I thought a month was a long time to get my first job after grad school, in a new country. The objective signs pointed to the fact I was on the right track. I was getting interviews for great positions. It was only my excessively high self-standards that were causing the anxiety. Looking back on this experience helps me anytime I'm feeling impatient about the pace of success.

To help ease any anxiety you may be feeling about the pace of your success, practice accepting that productivity and results can take time to come, and often come in cycles.

Experiment: Ask yourself the following questions:

1. Are there any areas of your life where you'd benefit from accepting the pace at which results and progress are occurring?

2. Is there objective evidence that suggests you are on the right track, and seeing positive results is merely a matter of patience and continuing to work methodically?

3. How would you talk to yourself differently if you had more acceptance of this? What would you say to yourself? Remember back to the self-compassion material from the last chapter. Flick back to that material if you need to refresh your memory or if you skipped that chapter.

Prevent Burnout by Navigating "I Just Need to Work Harder" Thoughts

Anxious perfectionists are often driven to work very hard by a swirly combination of ambition, conscientiousness, and fear that not going the extra mile will result in catastrophe. When something isn't going to plan, they can fall victim to the "I just need to work harder" thinking error.

This thinking error isn't solely the domain of anxious people. For example, it's one of the thinking errors that causes people to fail at diets over and over again. When someone flakes on a diet, that person usually jumps to the conclusion that the reason for the lack of success was not trying hard enough. The person vows to work harder but fails to put any strategies in place that, objectively, would likely result in more success. People who are sucked into this trap tend to keep trying failed strategies and expecting different results.

Here's an example of how I get pulled into this thinking trap and what I do to overcome it: I know from experience that aiming to write around 750 words a day is the sweet spot for me as a writing goal. When I set a higher number of words as my daily goal, I feel overwhelmed and end up procrastinating. I get less done overall. When things are going well, I usually stick to that minimum target. However, when I start to run out of energy, I have a tendency to *increase* the target because I'm feeling anxious about not getting enough done. To navigate this trap, all I need to do is recognize when I need to take a break for a day or two, but keep my goal consistent when I resume. I need to resist the urge to default to overworking when I'm feeling anxious or frustrated.

This pattern can be depicted as a set of flowcharts:

Trapped Pattern

Anxiety/frustration

⬇

"I need to work harder" thinking error

⬇

Increase my targets

⬇

Feel more anxious and possibly procrastinate

More Useful Pattern

Anxiety/frustration

"I need to work harder" thinking error

Spot the thinking trap

Take a break

Resume and maintain the behavioral goal
I know works for me

Experiment: Draw a flowchart that depicts one of your trapped patterns and a more useful pattern, just like I've done. The flowchart will show how your thoughts, feelings, and behaviors are connected. The general form to use is as follows; fill in the blanks.

Trapped Pattern

Anxiety/frustration

"I need to work harder" thinking error

Your unhelpful behavior pattern: _____

_____

More Useful Pattern

Anxiety/frustration

⬇

"I need to work harder" thinking error

⬇

Spot the thinking trap

⬇

A more useful behavior pattern: _____

_____

Being able to create your own cognitive behavioral flowcharts is an advanced psychological skill, but if you're keen to take up the challenge, it can be very helpful. Any of the material we cover in this book you can depict using flowcharts.

Navigate All-or-Nothing Thinking

Just like either/or thinking, all-or-nothing thinking is when you have difficulty seeing a middle ground. You either overdo things (all) or avoid them completely (nothing). For example, you might think that if you're going to start using social media, then you'll need to be on Facebook, Twitter, Pinterest, Instagram, and five other social networks. You either spread yourself too thin by pursuing all of them or feel overwhelmed and end up avoiding social media entirely.

Anxious perfectionists are especially prone to this trap, since anxiety makes people's thinking more rigid. When you choose the "nothing" option, your success rate slows because you're avoiding new things. Choosing the "all" option can lead to taking on too much, feeling exhausted, and making mistakes because you're tired. Catching this thinking error and learning to seek out the middle ground will go a long way to soothing your anxiety. The all-or-nothing trap is right up there with negative predictions as one of the key thinking biases for most anxious people.

Experiment: Are there any areas of your life right now where you're feeling anxious or overwhelmed because you've been overdoing something? Is there a middle ground option that you've previously been blind to?

We'll revisit this trap in Chapter 8 on avoidance.

Navigate "This Is Too Hard for Me" Thinking

Anxious perfectionists like to feel very on top of things. When they think, "This is too hard for me," they often treat it as fact, instead of recognizing it as potentially just another anxiety-induced false alarm. Remember, if you're anxiety-prone, then by definition your anxiety system is predisposed to false alarms— that is, registering dangers that aren't there.

Thoughts are just thoughts; the problem is that we accept thoughts as true, and confuse feelings with facts. Part of the reason this happens is memory bias: Your brain will tend to remember events from the past that match your current mood.[5] Because current mood has such a powerful effect on thoughts, consciously trying to recall evidence that you're skilled and talented probably won't feel very authentic or convincing when you're feeling down. If you know this is how your brain works, then you can discount some of the negative thoughts you have when you're in a deflated mood. Your thoughts will naturally improve when your mood improves. Therefore, regaining confidence is often just a matter of being patient and waiting for a negative or anxious mood to pass.

Experiment: Have there been any times in the past when you've had "this is too hard for me" thoughts, those thoughts have been a false alarm, and you've managed to do the thing you feared was too hard for you? Identify one example. Your example doesn't need to be something huge. A small example will do.

Shift Your View of What Constitutes a Good Idea

Anxious perfectionists often have sky-high expectations about what being good at generating ideas involves. They might think, "Since I didn't start a multibillion-dollar company in my garage by the time I was 21, then I'm obviously not an ideas person and am doomed to mediocrity." Does that sound excessively perfectionistic to you?

Excessive expectations plus anxiety get in the way of generating ideas. People get stuck in the ruminative thought, "Why can't I think of an idea?" Of course, this amplifies anxiety and makes it harder to think of anything. You might get stuck when generating ideas because you think you need to come up with something completely unique when, in reality, ideas are always built on other ideas. You can feel less frozen when it comes to generating ideas if you think of the process as retrieving information from your existing knowledge base.[6] If your sense is that generating ideas is like looking at a blank page, no wonder you're likely to have a freeze (or flee) anxiety reaction! Instead, try asking yourself:

- What do I know that's relevant to solving my problem or helping me answer my question?
- How could I replicate something I've already done successfully, but with a twist?
- How could I combine two concepts that could be combined but aren't usually? (Like croissants + donuts = cronuts)
- How could I take a successful method and replicate it with different ingredients? (Such as you notice the title of a viral blog post and copy the form of the title for a blog post you're writing about a different topic.)

Experiment: Try thinking of a successful method and how the method could be replicated but with different ingredients.

. . . .

Behavioral Shifts to Overcome Unhelpful Types of Perfectionism

Now that you're familiar with the common thinking biases that cause anxious perfectionists to get stuck, let's turn to behavioral tweaks that can help you stay calm, confident, and motivated.

Manage Your Willpower, Not Your Time

Anxious perfectionists often run their mental fuel tanks to empty, rather than keeping a little in reserve. When people act in ways that are inconsistent with their values and goals, it's typically because they've run out of willpower rather than out of time.

I like to think of willpower as being like computer RAM. RAM is the type of memory that your computer uses for running your programs and apps rather than the kind it uses to store your photos and documents. When you're running too many programs or apps at the same time, your system hangs and freezes. You need to make sure you always have a reserve of willpower available for on-the-fly decision making and controlling your reactions. If you run your willpower tank too low, you'll end up making poor choices or exploding at people. The following are some ways of making more willpower available to you:

- Reduce the number of tasks you attempt to get done each day to a *very* small number. Always identify what your most important task is, and make sure you get that single task done. You can group together your trivial tasks, like replying to emails or paying bills online, and count those as just one item.

- Refresh your available willpower by doing tasks slowly. My friend Toni Bernhard, author of *How to Wake Up: A Buddhist-Inspired Guide to Navigating Joy and Sorrow*, recommends doing a task 25% slower than your usual speed.[7] I'm not saying you need to do this all the time, just when you feel scattered or overwhelmed. Slowing down in this way is considered a form of mindfulness practice.

- Another way to refresh your willpower is by taking some slow breaths or doing any of the mindfulness practices from Chapter 5. Think of using mindfulness as running a cleanup on background processes that haven't shut down correctly. By using mindfulness to do a cognitive cleanup, you're not leaking mental energy to background worries and rumination.

- Reduce decision making. For many people, especially those in management positions or raising kids, life involves constant decision making. Decision making leeches willpower.[8] Find whatever ways you can to reduce decision making without it feeling like a sacrifice. Set up routines (like which meals you cook on particular nights of the week) that prevent you from needing to remake the same decisions over and over. Alternatively, outsource decision making to someone else whenever possible. Let other people make decisions to take them off your plate.

- Reduce excess sensory stimulation. For example, close the door or put on some dorky giant headphones to block out noise. This will mean your mental processing power isn't getting used up by having to filter out excess stimulation. This tip is especially important if you are a highly sensitive person (see Chapter 2 for more info if you skipped that chapter).

Know Your Warning Signs That You've Persisted Too Long

Because anxiety causes thinking to get narrow and rigid, it can sometimes cause you to persist too long on certain tasks. Since anxious perfectionists tend to be particular and don't like unfinished tasks hanging over their heads, they can be especially vulnerable to this trap. Know the signs that you need to stop persisting. For example, if you work online, one of your personal signs of overpersistence might be that you've searched a forum for over 30 minutes looking for a solution to a problem and haven't found it. This would be a cue that taking a break from trying to solve your problem is likely to be more effective than banging away at it. Another example might be if you've been trying to convince your partner of something for over 10 minutes. You've explained your point of view several different ways, and you're still at loggerheads.

Define your overpersistence warning signs in objective and specific ways. This will make it harder to ignore them than if your definitions were fuzzy.

Stop Midflow, Rather Than When You're Completely Exhausted or Stuck

As mentioned earlier, anxious perfectionists often run their will-power tanks to absolute empty. One way this manifests is by ceasing work only at the point when you're completely exhausted or stuck. This can make getting restarted on a task very unappealing, because your most recent memory of the task will be of it not going well or feeling exhausted while doing it. We all have *recency bias*, meaning recent memories tend to be the most salient. You don't want your most recent memory of a task to be of feeling stuck or wiped out from it.

Experiment with what it's like to stop working while you're in the zone and still enjoying a task rather than when you're exhausted and frustrated. Notice whether doing this leads to you making better subsequent choices. For example, better eating choices at night after a hard day.

Hand Over Control

If anyone has ever called you a control freak, recognize that your controlling ways and hesitancy about letting other people do things their way is likely to be anxiety related. Your thinking patterns may be related to fears that other people won't do tasks to a standard that's acceptable to you, which may or may not be true in any given instance. Or your controllingness might be related to "should" thinking errors, along the lines of "I should be able to do everything myself," or fears that needing help is a sign of being a weak person.

A behavioral experiment you can try is delegating or outsourcing tasks you feel overwhelmed by. For example, if you were a computer programmer and got stuck with an issue, you might put the problem you're stuck with on Odesk.com or a similar outsourcing platform, rather than persisting with trying to solve it yourself. Start by delegating smaller, less critical jobs, and see how it goes. Outsourcing tasks to others requires tolerating uncertainty and sometimes tolerating imperfect results. Try taking a big-picture perspective of whether outsourcing more tasks is a good investment overall.

If handing over tasks to others activates your difficulties in tolerating uncertainty, talk to yourself kindly about your feelings. Acknowledge that keeping a tight grip on the reins in every aspect of your life helps you feel secure but also acknowledge when that's wearing you out. Notice if being very controlling is one of those behavioral patterns that helps you feel less anxious in the short term but makes you feel more anxious in the long term. Being excessively controlling is one of those "the more you do it, the more you need to do it" anxiety patterns.

In Chapter 2, we discussed how care and caution can be helpful or can become excessive. Likewise, when it comes to being controlling, you might find it useful to distinguish between the types of maintaining control that are useful to you and those that aren't. This is a personal thing. For example, attempting to project-manage major home renovations might work for some people, but other people might become so stressed out by this that it puts a strain on their marriage. Again, it comes back to getting to know yourself.

Streamline Your Focus Instead of Jumping from Unfinished Project to Unfinished Project

Although it seems contradictory, anxiety-related perfectionism can cause people to persist too long on some tasks and leave other projects unfinished. Perfectionists who are intolerant of uncertainty often jump from project to project. They might start multiple business plans, grant proposals, job applications, movie scripts, stand-up routines, craft projects, or novels, and not finish any of them. They may sour quickly on an idea when their self-doubt starts to creep in rather than stay with the idea long enough to realistically judge it's potential.

If you bounce from idea to idea, it could very well be because it's hard for you to tolerate your uncertainty about whether the idea you're working on is going to pan out. If you have a habit of not finishing things, you're likely to be better off sticking with a project and finishing it, instead of jumping to another project when you start to feel unsure.

To help you be less tempted to jump around, reduce your exposure to excessive information and alternatives. For example, stop reading industry blogs for a while.

CHAPTER 7

....

Fear of Feedback and Criticism

How to Work with Your Sensitivity to Feedback

Feedback helps people improve, but anxious people often avoid it because it can feel threatening. Avoiding feedback due to anxiety may lead to slower than optimal progress in attaining your goals. Also, if you're closed off to feedback or react badly to it because of the anxiety it activates, your relationship with the feedback giver can become strained. This chapter will help you navigate these common issues.

Take the following quiz to see how this chapter pertains to you. Choose the answer that *best* applies. If no answer is the perfect fit, pick whichever is the closest.

1. You're considering getting feedback on work you've produced. How likely are you to expect that any feedback will be negative?

(A) I usually expect to get good feedback because I perceive myself as generally competent.

(B) I feel nervous about a negative response but not paralyzed by it.

(C) I tend to assume feedback will be negative.

2. When your boss points out nine things you're doing well and one valid area where you could improve, what's your typical reaction?

(A) I plan some simple actions that will ensure continued good feedback.

(B) I feel happy that the feedback was positive overall, but the negative comment irks me a little.

(C) The one negative comment bugs me for several days or more.

3. How confident are you in your ability to cope with valid negative feedback?

(A) I believe in my capacity to make necessary adjustments.

(B) I suspect I'd ruminate for a while, but I know I'd get through it after a quiet night in with a glass of wine and a Netflix marathon.

(C) I think I'd be so hurt and embarrassed I'd find it difficult to face the feedback giver if/when I see that person again.

4. How prone to personalizing negative feedback are you?

(A) I don't tend to personalize feedback.

(B) I personalize, but I have enough self-awareness that I usually catch myself doing it.

(C) When I get negative feedback, it feels like the person doesn't like me rather than doesn't like the work I've done.

5. How likely are you to avoid getting feedback on work you've produced?

(A) I don't avoid feedback; I see it as useful.

(B) I avoid feedback in some, but not all, areas of my life.

(C) I get feedback only if I absolutely have to; I'd rather go to the dentist.

6. When someone acts strangely toward you and there's no obvious reason why, what's your typical reaction?

(A) I think, "It could be about them rather than about me. Since I might never know the reasons behind the behavior, there's no point in overthinking it."

(B) I worry I've done something to offend the person, and I try to be extra nice and easygoing to fix the situation. The worry bothers me for a few days.

(C) It bothers me a great deal; I spend days thinking about what the reason for the person's behavior might have been.

7. **When you ask someone if you look fat in your jeans, do you really want to know the answer?**

(A) Yes.

(B) Yes, but I need the feedback giver to phrase their response delicately.

(C) Heck no.

Here's how to interpret your scores. If you scored:

Mostly A's

You generally think of feedback and criticism as helpful, and you're not threatened by it. If you feel a sting of disappointment when you get negative feedback, you're able to see this in context, without making a mountain out of a molehill. You perceive yourself as able to cope with feedback because you've done this successfully in the past. You're adept at taking feedback and making the necessary changes. You don't automatically jump to the conclusion that negative feedback means someone doesn't like you. You'll probably breeze through this chapter, but look out for any nuggets of new information.

Mostly B's

You're a bit prone to expecting that feedback will be negative. When you get mostly positive feedback with a few negatives thrown in, you tend to take the negatives to heart. While in many instances you can accept that feedback isn't personal, sometimes you get caught up in personalizing. There is a lot in this chapter that will help you feel more relaxed about feedback.

Mostly C's

Receiving feedback is extremely anxiety provoking for you. It makes you feel exposed and incredibly vulnerable. You expect that feedback will be negative and don't feel confident in your ability to fix problems highlighted by a feedback process. Negative feedback feels like a personal attack. You avoid getting feedback because it sends you into rumination mode and you find it difficult to break free. You're so fearful of feedback, you'll avoid opportunities if they will involve more exposure to it. You may never learn to love feedback, but the strategies in this chapter will help you become more comfortable and less avoidant.

This chapter isn't about completely turning off your sensitivity to criticism. It's about working with your natural sensitivity and learning to become less avoidant of feedback, even though it triggers feelings of vulnerability. You'll learn how to recognize thinking errors that might be amplifying your feedback fears, and you'll try experiments that will help you recognize when the benefits of getting outside input outweigh the discomfort.

. . . .

Thinking Shifts to Become More Relaxed About Feedback

The experiments in this section will help you understand your thinking processes around feedback and move your thoughts in a more balanced direction.

Fine-Tune Your Mind to the Benefits of Feedback

When you're in anxiety mode, it's easy to think of feedback as something wholly torturous and psychologically painful. Can you nudge this thinking by attuning to some of the benefits?

- You may find out you've done something well.
- You may discover that things you perceive as minor aspects of your work are seen by other people as major strengths.
- You may achieve more success because what you produce after feedback is better. For example, someone gives you a tip or suggests a change that improves your work. You realize you like the new version, but it wasn't something you would've attempted without a push in that direction.
- Through feedback, you may get new insights that help you solve problems you've been stuck with. The feedback giver may offer useful information about how he or she previously solved the problem you're currently having.
- Lastly, the process of receiving feedback can strengthen

your relationship with the person giving the feedback. It can be a bonding experience.

Experiment: Try one (or both) of these options:

Option 1: Think of one specific instance in the past when negative feedback has actually been useful to you.

Option 2: Go through each of the listed benefits of feedback, and write one example of a specific situation in which you received that benefit.

Recognize the Costs of Avoiding Feedback

When people avoid feedback, they miss out on benefits (covered earlier) and incur costs. For example, you might worry for longer than you need to about how your work will be perceived. Do you tend to think about the potential pain of getting feedback more than you think about the costs of avoiding it? If yes, you can consciously correct for this thinking bias. You might notice that this bias is another example of a principle we discussed earlier, in the chapter on hesitation: Anxious people tend to think about the potential harm of acting more than the potential harm of not acting.

Experiment: To get some big-picture perspective on what avoiding feedback has cost you, try answering the following questions. Write down one specific example of each. If you can't think of answers, let the questions marinate for a day or two.

- Have you avoided seeking feedback early on only to later realize that earlier feedback would've saved you from continuing down the wrong track for so long? When?
- Have you avoided feedback only to later realize your fears of negative feedback were unjustified? How long did you worry unnecessarily? What was that like for you?
- Have you had times when your predictions of negative feedback came true, but it was a much milder experience than you'd anticipated? Have you had an experience where you realized that making the required changes was much easier than you thought, and you had endured extra worry for no reason?
- What cool opportunities have you opted out of because you didn't want to expose yourself to even the possibility of negative feedback?

Correct Overestimated Feedback Fears

One of the reasons anxious people fear feedback is that they tend to judge their performance more harshly than others judge them.[1] If you're feeling anxious, you'll probably overestimate the likelihood that any feedback you'll get will be negative—the negative predictions thinking error.

Let's say you need to get feedback on your delivery of an upcoming presentation. You fear that you'll get crucified, that people will say your presentation style is horrible and won't say anything nice. How likely does this feared outcome feel? You might say, "It feels 99% likely." How likely is it in reality? You think, "Objectively, maybe 50%?" Your answer of 50% may still be an overestimate, but at least it jump-starts the shift in your thinking. It alerts you that your anxious feelings are, to some extent, clouding your perceptions.

Although it seems strange that people can shift their thinking just based on whether they are asked to think with their anxious mind or their objective mind, this isn't as far-fetched as it sounds. There's lots of research evidence that people's thinking changes based on how they're asked to think about something. For example, my own doctoral research asked people in relationships how their judgments of their romantic partner compared to reality. People recognized that they tended to view their partners more positively than warranted by reality.[2]

Experiment: Think of a current area in your life where feedback would be useful to you, but you're avoiding it. Ask yourself two questions (answer using a percentage, as shown in the example):

- How likely does it feel that I'm going to get very negative feedback?
- How likely is it in reality?

Believe in Your Ability to Cope with Negative Feedback

Just like everyone has a vision blind spot, everyone has cognitive blind spots that can lead to making less than stellar choices. For example, you think an outfit looks good on you, and in reality it doesn't. Or you thought you understood what your boss wanted but later realize you took the instructions in an unintended direction. Since we all have blind spots, making some mistakes and getting some negative feedback is unavoidable. Therefore, unless you plan to go live in a cave, you're going to need a game plan for how you'll cognitively and emotionally cope when negative feedback happens. We'll cover behavioral strategies later in the chapter, but let's work on the thinking and emotional aspects for now.

Experiment: Think about a specific scenario in which you fear negative feedback. If your fears came true:

- How would you go about making the required changes?
- How could you be self-accepting of your sensitivity to criticism? How could you talk to yourself gently about the emotions you're feeling instead of criticizing yourself for feeling upset? How could you be patient with yourself while you're having those feelings?
- What self-care would you do while you wait for your hurt and upset feelings to pass? (Yes, rewatching episodes of '90s TV is a totally acceptable answer.[3])
- What personal support would you access to cope with your emotions? For example, you'd talk to a friend.

Catch When You're Panicking About Ambiguous Feedback

Anxiety can cause people to sometimes misinterpret feedback once they've received it. When people feel anxious, they tend to interpret ambiguous information (and lack of feedback) as negative.[4] For example, your boss promises to get back to you in a couple of days about a request you've made. You assume this means the answer is going to be no. Another example: You might interpret lack of effusiveness in feedback as evidence the person wasn't impressed with your work. If the person just says "Thanks" when they'd usually say "Thanks, you did a great job," you interpret that as negative.

Experiment: Can you think of an example where you have jumped to a negative conclusion about ambiguous feedback or where you might be likely to do so?

Catch When You're Interpreting Negative Feedback as Worse Than It Is

There's also another way anxiety can cause people to misinterpret feedback they receive. If someone who is feeling anxious gets mildly negative feedback, that person often panics and sees it as much worse than it is. For example, you receive some comments on your work, and the first time you read them, the highlighted problems seem much more extensive than they will when you reread the feedback the next day.

Experiment: Can you think of a time when you've panicked upon receiving negative feedback and seen it as worse than it really was?

Minimize Personalizing of Feedback

We touched on personalizing in the chapter on rumination, but since personalizing feedback is a *very* common thinking error, let's briefly revisit it. I'm going to include being told no in response to requests under the feedback umbrella because getting a no answer can be considered a type of feedback. For example, you ask your boss if you can go to a conference and are told no. You take it personally, when, in reality, it has more to do with budgets.

Another example: You're not prone to speaking up, but you muster the courage to pitch an idea to your boss. She tells you she's "just not that into it." You feel crushed. Those negative feelings trigger panicky thoughts that your boss sees you as the least-smart person in the office, when you weren't having those thoughts previously.

There are two thinking shifts you need to make to overcome personalizing. The first is mindfulness: You need to train yourself to consider the possibility that whatever has happened might not be personal. The second is recognizing that negative feedback does not necessarily mean the person doesn't like you, doesn't respect your capabilities, or doesn't recognize your potential.

Experiment: Do you ever underestimate how capable and

talented others perceive you to be? Think of an example when you've possibly underestimated how positively you are perceived by someone.

Become Aware of Hostility Bias

Anxiety (and stress) can make people more vulnerable to the *hostility bias*, a type of personalizing where you jump to the conclusion that other people have hostile intent.[5] For instance, you hear people laughing and think they're laughing about you. For most people, this will just be a fleeting thought before they look around, check that their pants aren't on backward, and realize there's no possible reason the laughing could be about them.

The hostility bias often crops up in the workplace and in other group settings. For example, others offer you suggestions. You experience those suggestions as being attacked or nitpicked. You might have a combination of anxious thoughts and/or peeved off thoughts, such as, "Why are they being so pedantic?" Whether the peeved thoughts are justified or not is mostly irrelevant. What is relevant is that having these kinds of thoughts sometimes makes people feel very lonely, like it's them against the world.

Experiment: Can you think of any situations in which you're prone to hostility bias? For example, a coworker pointing out unimportant typos in your work. What are some alternative perspectives? Your coworker is trying to be helpful, or it's his issue—he's a bit OCD about typos.

When you experience the hostility bias, your feelings of anger can seem to go from 0 to 100 in two seconds flat. From an evolutionary perspective, anger is designed to make us act, not think. This makes it difficult to consider alternative thoughts when feeling angry. Therefore, the best way to tackle the hostility bias in the moment is to slow your breathing to calm yourself physiologically, then use a behavioral strategy such as "canned responses" (see the next section).

. . . .

Behavioral Shifts to Feel More Relaxed About Feedback

Use the following behavioral strategies in combination with the thinking shifts we've discussed to decrease your tendency to panic about feedback.

Develop Canned Responses to Feedback

You can prepare some verbal canned responses for times when you need to stall, without appearing defensive while you're mentally processing feedback. Some examples:

- I think you've got a good point about ____.
- I'll think about everything you've said. I need to process your feedback and mull it over.
- That's an interesting way to look at it.
- Let me think about how I can incorporate your feedback.

- Let me think about how best to proceed from here. I'll email you with some thoughts.

Canned responses should generally acknowledge any valid points the feedback giver has made and indicate you're going to go away and process the feedback. You can also have canned responses for when you feel embarrassed that a blind spot has been revealed. For example:

- I hadn't thought of it like that. That's really useful. Thanks for alerting me to that way of looking at it.
- That's a great idea. I often come away from our conversations with a new perspective.

If you have very high self-standards, you might need to act as if you are more self-accepting of having blind spots than you actually are!

Act As If You Feel Relaxed About Feedback

People sometimes feel a spike of defensiveness when they receive negative feedback. You might feel annoyed at the feedback or feel upset. In these situations, try acting as if you feel relaxed.[6] In other words, fake it till you make it. Acting as if you feel relaxed is one of the fastest ways to actually feel more calm. If you get an anxiety spike when you receive feedback or tend to feel defensive, try making your body language more open. Send nonverbal signals that you're open, even if inside you're not feeling it. Drop your shoulders, lift your head, make gentle eye contact, and relax your hands. When you do this, your thoughts and feelings will *start to* catch up with your nonverbal cues almost instantly. You won't feel completely relaxed, but it will help.

Consider Getting Your Own Supervision-Type Arrangement

People with anxiety are often most comfortable getting feedback one-on-one from someone who they're sure likes them and respects their talent.

A great way to achieve this is through a DIY supervision relationship. *Supervision* is a term psychologists and counselors use for having regular meetings with a colleague, usually once a fortnight or once a month. During the meetings, supervisees talk to their supervisors about the thinking processes they've used to make complex decisions. Supervisees sometimes also discuss how personal issues might be influencing their work and how to prevent any potential harm from this. *Supervision* is a bit of a funny term because even psychologists who've been practicing for decades still do it. This tradition is based on the idea that all of us have cognitive blind spots, regardless of our level of experience and talent. The supervisor generally isn't the supervisee's direct manager. They're usually someone who is external to the organization where the supervisee works, or a senior colleague.

A difference between supervision and mentoring is that

supervision is aimed at making sure therapists are doing the absolute best work possible with their clients. In other words, it's for the benefit of the clients rather than for the benefit of the therapist. Consider whether your job would potentially allow you to undertake a supervision-type scenario during your working hours. If you frame it as supervision, aimed at benefiting your current work rather than as about your general career development, you may have more luck in convincing your boss.

When you practice exposing yourself to feedback from someone who you know respects your abilities, it will help you build up your tolerance for feedback so you avoid it less. This setup will also allow you to experiment with being more real, vulnerable, and honest about any stuck points you may be having in your job that are getting in the way of optimal productivity and decision making.

Practice the Poop Sandwich

When you ask people to give you feedback, ask for it in the form of a "poop sandwich." The poop sandwich is feedback given in the following order—something you did well, a problem or learning edge, something else you did well. Try to give and receive feedback using this technique. The bread in the sandwich (the positives) needs to be genuine for the poop sandwich to be effective. The poop sandwich concept is cheesy, but almost all of us find it easier to listen to feedback when we get a little validation first.

Get a Very Small Sample of Feedback

Sometimes anxious people need time to process a little bit of feedback before they're open to receiving more. For example, if you're developing a website, you might do some initial user testing with one to three people.

If you find you need time to lick your wounds after receiving negative feedback, be kind to yourself about this. Getting a small sample of feedback is a great way to learn via experience that you can cope with feedback and that it helps to treat yourself kindly throughout the process.

CHAPTER 8

....

Avoidance

How to Stop Putting Your Head
in the Sand About Important Things

We covered hesitating when you want to do something way back in Chapter 4. Now, we'll address avoiding things you need to do but would much rather not do.

Take the following quiz to see how this chapter pertains to you. Choose the answer that *best* applies. If no answer is the perfect fit, pick whichever is the closest.

1. What do you do when you feel intimidated by an important task?

(A) Identify part of the task I don't feel intimidated by and start with that.

(B) Put off the task for a while but eventually get around to it.

(C) Permanently stuff the task into my overflowing "too-hard" basket.

2. How much time do you spend doing activities that other people might describe as a waste of time?

   (A) An amount of time that helps me refresh.

   (B) Enough time that I regret it, but not so much time that it interferes with completing important tasks.

   (C) So much time that it interferes with getting critical tasks done.

3. How often do you work on low-priority tasks because your higher-priority tasks feel outside your comfort zone?

   (A) Rarely.

   (B) Occasionally.

   (C) You can often find me fiddling with the font on a document.

4. Does anyone ever get annoyed with you due to your avoidance of tasks or issues? For example, your spouse gets frustrated that you put off making phone calls that you feel anxious about.

   (A) No.

   (B) Not overtly, but if asked, my family and/or coworkers would probably say it bugs them that I procrastinate, opt out of some activities, or ignore necessary tasks.

   (C) Yes, it's a topic of conflict.

5. **What do you do when you need to do something that brings up memories of prior failures or bad past experiences?**

(A) Adopt a growth mindset; I can improve through the right kinds of practice.

(B) Do the task if I absolutely have to but avoid it if I have any choice.

(C) Avoid doing it even when that could create problems; for example, I would avoid calling a plumber to deal with an issue if the last time I dealt with a plumber was a bad experience.

6. **What do you do when you're working on a joint project and you need to raise an issue about someone else's work?**

(A) Decide whether a direct or subtle approach is likely to be best in the specific situation.

(B) Drop hints and hope the person gets the message.

(C) Do nothing, or complain to everyone except the person whose work is at issue.

Here's how to interpret your scores. If you scored:

Mostly A's

Avoidance coping isn't a major issue for you. You can deal with difficult thoughts and feelings without avoiding important tasks. You're willing to withstand some feelings of anxiety and worry to take care of things that need doing. You'll probably move quickly through this chapter. Expect to learn a few nuggets of new info for yourself and to better understand other people in your life for whom avoidance is an issue.

Mostly B's

Some room for improvement. You don't avoidance-cope to the extent that your life is a mess (for example, you file your tax return on time), but you tend to limit yourself to things that are within your comfort zone, which can cause problems for you sometimes. You avoid anxiety-provoking interpersonal situations, like difficult conversations with employers, coworkers, or friends. The tips in this chapter will help you move your answers from B's to A's.

Mostly C's

You're caught in the awful, self-perpetuating cycle of avoiding things that feel stressful, but then that avoidance creates extra stress in the long run. Your avoidance is probably causing you to feel stuck or paralyzed in your life overall. There is a lot in this chapter that will help you reduce your avoidance coping and therefore reduce your overall stress.

Avoidance is one of the main factors that fuels anxiety.[1] Avoidance can be behavioral—you avoid situations or doing things that make you feel anxious. Or it can be cognitive—you try to avoid thinking about topics that trigger your anxiety.

Avoidance will eat you alive psychologically if you don't work on it. Avoidance coping generates additional stress in your life.[2] Further, the more you avoid, the more your anxiety will tend to spread to other tasks and situations. And when you avoid, you miss out on opportunities to learn that you can cope with situations, and you miss out on gaining skills through experience.

In this chapter, you'll learn about the psychological mechanisms that underlie avoidance, and learn thinking and behavioral strategies for scaling it back. Since overcoming avoidance is hard, expect that your progress in this area might feel a bit like two steps forward, one step backward. However, even with this pattern of imperfect progress, you can expect to feel a lot better overall.

· · · · · · · · · · · · ·

Thinking Shifts to Overcome Avoidance

This section will help you understand your patterns of avoidance coping and show you how thinking shifts can increase your belief in your ability to cope with whatever it is you're avoiding.

Know Yourself: Are You a Freezer, Flyer, or Fighter?

How avoidance coping manifests for you will depend on what your dominant response type is when you're facing something you'd rather avoid. There are three possible responses: freezing, fleeing, or fighting. We've evolved these reactions because they're useful for encounters with predators. Like other animals, when we encounter a predator, we're wired to freeze to avoid provoking attention, run away, or fight.

Most people are prone to one of the three responses more so than the other two. Therefore, you can think of yourself as having a "type," like a personality type. Identify your type using the descriptions in the paragraphs that follow. Bear in mind that your type is just your most dominant pattern. Sometimes you'll respond in one of the other two ways.

Freezers virtually freeze when they don't want to do something. They don't move forward or backward; they just stop in their tracks. If a coworker or loved one nags a freezer to do something the freezer doesn't want to do, the freezer will tend not to answer. Freezers may be prone to *stonewalling* in relationships, which is a term used to describe when people flat-out refuse to discuss certain topics that their partner wants to talk about, such as a decision to have another baby or move to a new home.[3]

Flyers are people who are prone to fleeing when they don't want to do something. They might physically leave the house if a relationship argument gets too tense and they'd rather not continue the discussion. Flyers can be prone to serial relationships because they'd rather escape than work through tricky issues. When flyers want to avoid doing something, they tend to busy themselves with too much activity as a way to justify their avoidance. For example, instead of dealing with their own issues, flyers may overfill their children's schedules so that they're always on the run, taking their kids from activity to activity.

143

Fighters tend to respond to anxiety by working harder. Fighters are the anxiety type that is least prone to avoidance coping; however, they still do it in their own way. When fighters have something that they'd rather not deal with, they will often work themselves into the ground but avoid dealing with the crux of the problem. When a strategy isn't working, fighters don't like to admit it and will keep hammering away. They tend to avoid getting the outside input they need to move forward. They may avoid acting on others' advice if doing so is anxiety provoking, even when deep down they know that taking the advice is necessary. Instead, they will keep trying things their own way.

A person's dominant anxiety type—freezer, flyer, or fighter—will often be consistent for both work and personal relationships, but not always.

Experiment: Once you've identified your type, think about a situation you're facing currently in which you're acting to type. What's an alternative coping strategy you could try? For example, your spouse is nagging you to do a task involving the computer. You feel anxious about it due to your general lack of confidence with all things computer related. If you're a freezer, you'd normally just avoid answering when asked when you're going to do the task. How could you change your reaction?

Use a Values Conflict to Overcome Avoidance

People usually think of guilt as a negative emotion. However, research has shown that feeling guilt tends to be associated with taking others' perspectives and positive behaviors, such as genuine apologies and making amends.[4] If you can recognize how avoidance coping contradicts your values, you can use the ensuing healthy guilt to your advantage.

For example, your value may be "Do unto others." Yet you've been avoiding telling someone that you're going to deny a request she's made. Imagine the shoe on the other foot: If you were waiting on a response from someone, wouldn't you rather be told as soon as possible so you could make other plans? By recognizing the gap between your values and your behavior, you can find the motivation to overcome your avoidance.

Note: Guilt is psychologically healthy. Shame is not. The difference between guilt and shame is that guilt is about feeling bad about a behavior; shame is about feeling bad about who you are.[5] Self-criticism usually involves inducing shame.

Experiment: Identify a situation where your avoidance contradicts your values. How could you resolve your values–behavior conflict?

Use a Growth Mindset to Overcome Avoidance

Let's look at how having a fixed mindset can drive avoidance coping, and how a growth mindset can overcome it. You may want to turn back to Chapter 4 for a refresher on fixed vs. growth mindsets. Consider a commonly avoided behavior: investing. What might someone who has a fixed mindset about investing think? That person might think something like "I don't understand investing. It's all over my head. It's just not something I can grasp. I'm doomed to make mistakes with my investing choices."

What would a person with a growth mindset think? It would be more like "I can probably find some information that's designed to help people like me. With a bit of practice and perseverance, I'll learn to distinguish between reliable and unreliable information and make good decisions."

Experiment: Identify the area of your life where avoidance is creating the *most* serious problems. Write out fixed and growth mindset perspectives like the examples just given.

Recognize That Knowing Is Better Than Not Knowing

In the last chapter, we discussed how people avoid feedback when they lack confidence in their ability to correct problems highlighted by the feedback process. More generally, people tend to avoidance-cope when they fear getting negative information and they're not confident they could cope with that effectively. They'd rather keep their head in the sand. If you up your belief in your ability to cope with facing an upsetting reality, you'll experience less desire to avoid.

Let's say you're avoiding retirement planning because you fear learning that the amount you'd need to save to have a comfortable retirement is unachievable. If this happened, how would you cope? Would you take to your bed and never get up? No, you wouldn't. You'd likely do a mix of behavioral coping (changing your spending and investing patterns) and emotional coping, such as giving yourself self-compassion for mistakes you've made in the past.

Experiment: Identify an example of your avoidance coping that's driven by fear you'd be unable to cope with facing facts. Imagine vividly and specifically what you'd do. You can do this as a three-minute writing experiment or just think it through. What's a possible new thought that recognizes your ability to cope? For example, "If I start addressing my debt, I might feel overwhelmed with anxiety for a period, but then I'll figure out a way forward, and my financial anxiety will become easier to cope with."

Catch the Thought Distortions Underlying Procrastination

Procrastination is something we all do, but anxiety and a pattern of avoidance coping can cause procrastination to get out of hand. The good and bad news is that the same old thinking errors that have come up in previous chapters are also the thinking patterns that underlie procrastination. Even though the concepts are simple in theory, thinking errors are sneaky and can be hard to spot. They're like shapeshifters who show up in different manifestations. To go beyond a surface level of understanding, people usually need to hear examples related specifically to the situations they're facing. Therefore, even though we've covered these already, you can never have too many examples. When you find yourself procrastinating, run through this list of thinking errors to see if any of them are contributing. When you identify the thinking error you're making, it will help you identify a behavioral way forward that feels achievable.

Experiment: Place a check mark in the right-hand column if you sometimes procrastinate due to these thinking biases. Once you're done, identify one task you're currently avoiding where one of these thinking errors is playing a role. Choose an alternative, more useful thought.

Thinking Bias	Examples	That's Me (indicate with a ✓)
All or nothing thinking / Rigid thinking / Unrelenting standards / Perfectionism	• You need to clean a whole room but don't have the energy. You do nothing rather than clean one or two things in the room.	❑
	• You believe that everything needs to be done to an excellent level. If you can't do something to an excellent level, you tend to avoid it completely.	❑
	• You set unrealistic productivity goals for how much you can get done. This causes you to avoid everything completely because you feel overwhelmed.	❑
Negative predictions	• You expect that if you try something you'll fail.	❑
	• You put off asking for things because you think other people won't be interested or expect they'll say no (mind reading).	❑
	• You put off getting user feedback because you expect it will be negative / You avoid testing products with real customers.	❑
	• You overestimate how difficult or unpleasant a task will be.	❑
Underestimating your ability to cope	• You underestimate your ability to cope with boring, stressful, or anxiety-provoking tasks.	❑

Thinking Bias	Examples	That's Me (indicate with a ✓)
Personalizing: personalizing your difficulty with a task rather than seeing the task itself as difficult, which gives you an excuse to avoid	• You think the reason you struggle with something is because you're too stupid to figure it out rather than thinking it's inherently challenging and has a learning curve.	❑
	• You think you're the only one who has problems with something.	❑

• • • • • • • • • • • •

Behavioral Shifts to Overcome Avoidance Coping

Thinking shifts are only half the answer when it comes to stopping avoidance coping. You have to marry your thinking shifts with little shifts in your behavior. The more tiny behavioral shifts you make to scale back your avoidance, the less you'll experience urges to avoid in the first place. In other words, your behavior will influence your thoughts and feelings. The strategies in this section, combined with the thinking shifts we've discussed, will help you make significant changes in your avoidance habits.

Work Through a Hierarchy of Avoided Situations

Back in Chapter 5 on rumination, we covered imagery exposure. Let's now talk about a different type of exposure technique. Virtually every version of CBT for anxiety disorders involves working through what's called an *exposure hierarchy*. The concept is simple. You make a list of all the situations and behaviors you avoid due to anxiety. You then assign a number to each item on your list based on how anxiety provoking you expect doing the avoided behavior would be. Use numbers from 0 (= not anxiety provoking at all) to 100 (= you would fear having an instant panic attack). For example, attempting to talk to a famous person in your field at a conference might be an 80 on the 0–100 scale.

Sort your list in order, from least to most anxiety provoking. Aim to construct a list that has several avoided actions in each 10-point range. For example, several that fall between 20 and 30, between 30 and 40, and so on, on your anxiety scale. That way, you won't have any jumps that are too big. Omit things that are anxiety provoking but wouldn't actually benefit you (such as eating a fried insect).

Make a plan for how you can work through your hierarchy, starting at the bottom of the list. Where possible, repeat an avoided behavior several times before you move up to the next level. For example, if one of your items is talking to a colleague you find intimidating, do this several times (with the same or different colleagues) before moving on.

When you start doing things you'd usually avoid that are low on your hierarchy, you'll gain the confidence you need to do the things that are higher up on your list. It's important you don't use what are called *safety behaviors*. Safety behaviors are things people do as an anxiety crutch—for example, wearing their lucky undies when they approach that famous person or excessively rehearsing what they plan to say.

There is a general consensus within psychology that exposure techniques like the one just described are among the most effective ways to reduce problems with anxiety. In clinical settings, people who do exposures get the most out of treatment.[6] Some studies have even shown that just doing exposure can be as effective as therapies that also include extensive work on thoughts.[7] If you want to turbocharge your results, try exposure. If you find it too difficult to do alone, consider working with a therapist.

Try a 30-Day Project for Overcoming Avoidance Coping

Avoidance coping habits aren't something you can snap your fingers and change. A 30-day project focused on gradually turning around avoidance coping can help. You can use this approach as an alternative to the exposure hierarchy if doing a 30-day project seems more appealing or relevant to you.

During the 30 days, take as many opportunities as you can to be less avoidant than you usually would be. This will help you overcome any problems you might have with not knowing where to start in reducing your avoidance. As situations come up, focus on taking some action, even if you're not certain what the absolute right action is. For example, if you're confused by all the options for backing up your digital photos in the cloud, you might ask your most tech-savvy friend what she does, and just go with that. You can always switch later.

Don't be too all-or-nothing about overcoming avoidance coping. We all have only so much willpower available for dealing with things we'd prefer not to do. The goal is to start unraveling your avoidance coping habits bit by bit. If you sometimes fall back into the avoidance coping trap, that's to be expected.

Next Action

When you're avoiding something, try identifying the next action you need to take to move forward. Do that action. For example, if you have a legal situation and you feel overwhelmed about it, the next action you need to take might be something like emailing a lawyer friend and asking for a referral. If your garden has become overgrown with weeds, the next action you need to take might be locating your gardening tools. If your smartphone is acting up, the next action you need to take might be to run a backup. If you need to buy a new laptop, your next action might be to decide on your budget. Keep in mind that the next action you pick shouldn't be too big. Generally, try to think of something you can do in 15 minutes or less. If you still feel overwhelmed, try picking an even smaller next action. To give credit where credit is due, the concept of defining your next action was first popularized in a productivity book called *Getting Things Done.*[8] It's a concept many of my clients have found useful.

Use Technology to Overcome Avoidance

There are many technology solutions that can help you overcome avoidance. While you probably don't want to spend a lot of time investigating these or setting them up, using a handful of these solutions may work well for you. Here are some examples:

- If you usually mull over how to respond to emails for longer than is useful, try deciding to respond sooner and write shorter replies. Sign up for Gmail and enable the "undo send" setting so that you have 30 seconds to unsend an email.[9] It's remarkable how this 30 seconds is usually long enough to catch important things you either forgot to say or want to phrase differently.
- You can use an app for your web browser to lock yourself out of certain websites after a set number of minutes of use. For example, you might use this to limit Facebook to a half hour a day (see TheAnxietyToolkit.com/resources for app suggestions).
- If you have a small business but you're not good at keeping receipts for business expenses, you can use an app that will automagically create receipts for your small purchases,

based on importing your credit card statement (again, see TheAnxietyToolkit.com/resources for details).

Try thinking of two or three apps that, if they existed, would be very helpful to you. Chances are they do exist! Once you know what problem you need to solve, you can find the app that's the best fit for your needs. Lifehacker.com is an example of a website that you can use to find the apps you're after.

Blitz Small Avoided Tasks

Because it's easy to run out of willpower for nonurgent tasks, they can mount up. For example, you might have unwanted magazine subscriptions, credit cards you don't use that are incurring a fee, or other services that need to be canceled. If you have tasks like this that will take less than 15 minutes each to take care of, you may want to blitz two or three of them at once. Think about when you're likely to have the time and willpower available for doing this. Schedule when and where you plan to do it. Make sure you're being realistic about how much time taking care of each item will require. Also, don't mix together avoided tasks that will take a long time and those that can be dealt with quickly. Blitz just the small ones. An alternative to blitzing several tasks at once would be to make a list and then commit to doing one quick (less than 15 minutes) task each day. Experiment with which approach works best for you.

Reward Yourself

After you've worked on a task you've been avoiding, allow yourself to enjoy the fruits of your labor by taking some time to relax. This might be as simple as working on cleaning out a cupboard one evening and then savoring an episode of your favorite TV show afterward. Behaviors that get rewarded are more likely to persist. Therefore, by rewarding yourself, you're making it more likely that you'll tackle avoided tasks in the future.

Pick rewards that really are rewards. A supersize portion of fries that you're going to regret later isn't a reward. A general psychological principle is that rewards work best when there is a natural fit between the reward and the behavior being rewarded. Since avoidance coping involves putting off hard things, it makes sense to reward yourself with relaxation after tackling things you've been avoiding.

If tackling avoidance results in saving a sum of money, then you might allow yourself to spend some of that money in another area that's of more value to you. If you cancel a $50-a-year subscription that you're not actually using, then you might allow yourself to purchase something you've been wanting up to that value. It's a natural consequence that if you spend less in one area, you'll have more to spend in other areas, so this reward would be a good natural fit.

Practice Doing Scaled-Down Versions of Tasks

As a behavioral experiment, try doing a simpler version of something you've been putting off. While chipping away is sometimes necessary, where possible, shrink the task rather than just spreading it out. Personalize the task in a way that meets your needs, preferences, and the amount of time/money/energy/willpower you have available. Some examples will show you exactly what I mean.

Big Version	Easier Version	Easiest Version
Make a schedule for your time use.	Make a schedule for part of each day, such as the morning.	Before leaving work each day, schedule one task for the following day.
Redo your kitchen.	Change your kitchen cabinets.	Paint your cabinets.
Do 20 minutes of meditation each day.	Do three minutes of mindful walking each day.	Take one mindful breath before getting out of bed each morning.
Monitor all your spending.	Monitor your spending in the area where you tend to overspend the most, such as groceries.	Monitor how many times you go to Whole Foods each week.

Note that I'm not saying the scaled-down examples are better choices than the comprehensive versions. It's just that sometimes the best option requires too much willpower to implement. Therefore, look for the best choice for the amount of willpower you have available to spend. Using a framework like the one shown in the table guides you to think of your choices in terms of a limited set of alternatives and therefore helps you overcome choice overload. Tweak the framework if you want to personalize it.

As we covered in Chapter 4, you should assume that if you don't plan when and where you're going to do something, you're probably not going to do it. If you avoid choosing when and where you'll do a task, take that as a clue that you're not committed to doing it. Most likely, you're biting off something that is bigger than the willpower you currently have available. Pick a smaller action for which you are willing to plan when and where you'll do it.

Adopt a Flexible Approach to Reducing Procrastination

Procrastination isn't always a bad thing.[10] Sometimes the urge to procrastinate is a cue that you need a mental break, so that when you restart a task, you're refreshed and more productive. However, if you think procrastination is a problem for you, try these principles:

- Take breaks after you've done some work, not before.
- If you're going to procrastinate, at least procrastinate by doing something useful. Do an avoided task that's slightly more appealing than whatever task you're most keen to avoid. Thinking back to high school or college, you may

remember how cleaning your room all of a sudden became much more appealing when you were supposed to be studying for exams.

- Antiprocrastination strategies that can work well for a while can stop working. Accept that you'll need to switch strategies in and out. For example, you may find that putting a clean set of gym clothes in your car before you go to bed each night makes you more likely to go to the gym the next day. However, this might work for only a couple of months before you start skipping the gym again. When this happens, switch up your strategies. Maybe you need to try another type of exercise. Maybe the problem is that you're too busy at work and therefore don't have any willpower available for the gym. If this is the case, you'd want to solve the problem at its source—by reducing your willpower drain at work.

PART 3

Where to Next?

CHAPTER 9

. . . .

Managing Your Anxiety vs. Living Your Life

Through Parts 1 and 2 of this book, you've been intensively focusing on building your Anxiety Toolkit. This chapter will guide you toward how you can consolidate and improve your skills over the coming months, without feeling like you've become your own full-time psychologist!

Take the following quiz to see how this chapter pertains to you. Choose the answer that *best* applies. If no answer is a perfect fit, pick whichever is the closest.

1. **How easy does it feel to integrate your Anxiety Toolkit skills into your everyday life?**

   (A) As easy as integrating ice cream into my everyday life would be. I don't feel overburdened by it.

   (B) It feels OK, but I could simplify it more.

   (C) It feels like a lot of work.

2. **How clear are you on which cognitive biases are the most important for you to keep working on going forward?**

   (A) That's easy. I know what my most common thinking traps are.

   (B) I have an understanding of what my common thinking traps are, but I haven't prioritized them yet.

   (C) I haven't thought about that yet.

3. **Do you catch your thinking errors at the time, or only long after the fact?**

   (A) Usually the same day the thinking error occurs. For example, I might realize while driving home from work that I had personalized feedback during the day.

   (B) A mixture—sometimes at the time, but sometimes not until long after something has happened.

   (C) I tend to recognize my thinking errors only when I'm reading anxiety materials or talking to a therapist.

4. **How clear are you on which anxiety-related behavior patterns are the most important for you to keep working on? For example, avoidance coping.**

   (A) That's easy—I know which of the behavior patterns that we've covered are the biggest issues for me.

(B) My list is too long. I need to narrow it down to the behavior patterns that are my biggest issues.

(C) Darn, I haven't thought about that yet.

5. **Do you have routines in your life that keep your anxiety engine running cool and help prevent it from being too reactive?**

(A) Yes, I exercise and do some of the mindfulness meditations from the rumination chapter.

(B) Sort of. I'm a bit hit or miss with my routines.

(C) No, not really.

6. **How manageable do you find your routines for keeping your anxiety engine cool?**

(A) Very manageable—they're as much a standard part of my day as brushing my teeth.

(B) Honestly, if I got busy, I might start skipping them.

(C) They still feel too much like hard work.

Here's how to interpret your scores. If you scored:

Mostly A's
Nice job. It seems like you've mostly figured out how to integrate your Anxiety Toolkit skills into your everyday life.

You're clear what you need to focus on most, from both a thinking and a behavioral traps perspective. You're likely to be most interested in the section of this chapter on broadening your cognitive behavioral skills beyond those that relate directly to anxiety. Congratulations on the hard work you've done so far.

Mostly B's

You're almost in good shape. You've been following along with the core concepts, but now is the time to consolidate and simplify which Anxiety Toolkit skills to focus on going forward. This chapter will help you get a laser focus on where you're at and which thinking and behavioral traps are the most important for you to keep in mind as you go about your life.

Mostly C's

When people take on a big project, like a major home renovation or learning cognitive behavioral skills, things usually get really messy and unwieldy before everything comes together. You're still at the messy stage. That's OK. This chapter will help you move on from that stage and move from C's to A's.

When people come to therapy for anxiety disorders, the treatment period typically lasts three to six months. After that point, it's usually good for people to try using their skills on their own.

If you've been working on your anxiety intensively for a period of time, and you've experienced some insights and improvements, then it's probably time to take a break from such an intensive focus. This chapter, and the two that follow it, will help you achieve a balance between continuing to practice the Anxiety Toolkit skills you've been learning and getting on with living your life. You can continue to pay attention to catching and countering your thinking errors and anxiety-related behavior patterns, but let that move to the background.

. . . .

Moving Your Anxiety to a Secondary Focus

Here are some ways to begin moving your anxiety to a background focus in your life.

Simplify Your Focus

We've covered many different types of thinking errors and behavioral traps. Most people get caught in all of them from time to time, but there are likely to be a handful that are the biggest issues for you. For example, negative predictions (expecting negative outcomes) and all-or-nothing thinking tend to be the two most common thinking traps for people. Try identifying your two most common thinking errors and your two most common anxiety-related behavioral traps from those we've discussed. The behavioral patterns on your list might include things like overworking to try to relieve anxiety, avoidance coping when you feel anxious, or hesitating too long before acting when you feel uncertain.

When you feel high anxiety or feel stuck and you're trying to find a way forward, first look to see if any of your most common patterns is playing a role. Try coming up with alternative, more balanced thoughts and behaviors. If none of your top four seems to be the problem, then you can look more widely at the other traps we've covered to understand what might be going on.

Weekly Check-Ins

Instead of focusing on your anxiety all the time, try scheduling a weekly check-in session with yourself. Clients who have been coming to sessions weekly often just put that same day and time aside. Instead of meeting with me, they meet with themselves. You can do the same.

Pick a time and place that will work for you to do your weekly check-in. Start a notebook (or use the note-taking app on your phone) in which you can record things you might want to address during your weekly check-in. When it comes time for your check-in, use the list as your agenda. If you have lots of issues that come up during the week and end up with a long agenda, just pick the one or two that seem most important to work through.

This process will allow you to take some time to focus on any anxiety-driven issues that occurred during the week that you didn't get a chance to deal with as they happened or where you tried something but it didn't seem to do the trick. Remember to include behavioral traps, like overworking or avoidance coping, if these have occurred during the week.

For each issue, go back to what seems like the most relevant chapter and try a solution from that chapter. For example, if you noticed yourself ruminating about a problem but didn't take problem-solving action (meaning you didn't move from thinking about the problem to taking a behavioral action), you might try defining your problem, generating a list of your best three to six options for moving forward with that problem, picking one option, and planning when and where you're going to implement that solution.

Plans, Hobbies, and Working Out

Now is a great time to shift your focus to new plans, hobbies, or interests.

What is something you've been putting off due to anxiety that you'd like to focus on in the upcoming months? It could be anything from dating, to weekly dinners with friends, to starting an investment plan, to searching for a job that you think would be a better fit for you than your current job.

Now's also a good time to think about getting moving. Exercise has natural antidepressant and anti-anxiety qualities.[1] I don't want to labor the point because we've all heard about the importance of exercise a million and one times already. However, it would be remiss of me not to mention exercise as an anxiety antidote. For many people, it's easier to exercise if they focus on the mental health benefits of exercise rather than the physical health benefits. Why? You get the mental health benefits from exercise more or less straightaway, whereas for some of the physical benefits, you might not reap those until you're older.

Here's a tip for why anxious people sometimes delay making an exercise plan: Anxious people who dislike uncertainty sometimes get frozen on pause because of all the conflicting information about exactly how much exercise they should do and at what intensity. The bottom line: Incorporate exercise into your life however you can. Assuming you're doing it safely and are in good physical health, doing any exercise at all is always going to be better than not doing any.

Practice Mindfulness Meditation

Mindfulness meditation, which might be just a slow breathing routine, helps many people manage their anxiety. This can be as simple as taking one slow breath before you get out of bed, doing four to six slow breaths when you notice yourself feeling an anxiety spike, or doing a daily three minutes of any of the mindfulness meditations from the rumination chapter. If/when you get bored with your mindfulness or exercise routines, change them up.

Set Up Your Life to Suit Your Temperament

Way back in Chapter 2, we talked about how people differ from one another in terms of qualities like their preferred level of sociability and how much psychological energy it takes them to adapt to change. When the routines and circumstances of your life are set up so that your lifestyle is a good fit for your natural preferences, it can give you a feeling of being in equilibrium. This will help prevent you from getting overwhelmed by anxiety on a regular basis. And by arranging your life to suit your temperament, you'll have the time to process and calm down from life events that make you feel anxious. Some areas in which you can set up your life to fit your temperament are:

- Have the right level of busyness in your life. For example, have enough after-work or weekend activities to keep you feeling calmly stimulated but not overstimulated and scattered. Note that being understimulated (for example, having too few enjoyable activities to look forward to) can be as much of a problem as being overstimulated.
- Pick the physical activity level that's right for you. Fine-tuning your physical activity level could be as simple as getting up from your desk and taking a walk periodically to keep yourself feeling calm and alert. Lifting things (such as carrying shopping bags up stairs) can also increase feelings of alertness and energy. Having pleasurable activities to look forward to and enough physical activity will help protect you against depression.
- Have the right level of social contact in your life, and have routines that put this on autopilot. For example, a routine of having drinks after work on a Friday with friends, or attending a weekly class with your sister. Achieving the right level of social contact might also include putting

mechanisms in place to avoid too much social interruption, like having office hours rather than an open-door policy.

- Keep a balance of change and routine in your life. For example, alternate going somewhere new for your vacation vs. returning to somewhere you know you like. What the right balance of change and routine is for you will depend on your natural temperament and how much change vs. stability feels good to you.

- Allow yourself the right amount of mental space to work up to doing something—enough time that you can do some mulling over the prospect of getting started but not so much time that it starts to feel like avoidance of getting started.

- If coping with change sucks up a lot of energy for you, be patient with yourself, especially if you're feeling stirred up by change or a disruption to your routines or plans. As mentioned in Chapter 2, keep some habits and relationships consistent when you're exploring change in other areas.

- Have self-knowledge of what types of stress you find most difficult to process. Don't voluntarily expose yourself to those types without considering alternatives. For example, if you want a new house and you know you get stressed out by making lots of decisions, then you might choose to buy a house that's already built, rather than building your own home. If you know making home-improvement decisions is anxiety provoking for you, you might choose to move to a house that's new or recently renovated, rather than doing any major work on your current home or buying a fixer-upper. There's always a balance with avoidance coping, where some avoidance of the types of stress that you find most taxing can be very helpful.

Reaching Out

When you've been looking inward for a period of time, it's good to switch that up and spend some time focusing outward on your relationships with others. It's sometimes easy to forget other people's emotional needs when you're putting so much hard work into your own. For example, if you have a spouse or partner (or child), what are his or her emotional needs right now? What kind of nurturing and encouragement does he or she need from you? I'm not necessarily suggesting anything hugely elaborate here: Maybe you've gotten out of the habit of kissing hello and good-bye each day. Maybe your spouse makes some of the same thinking errors that you do, and you could work on them together.

If you have a spouse or partner, ask what nurturing and encouragement he or she needs from you now and in the coming months. If you don't get a clear answer, then try focusing on how you say good-bye and hello each day. For most couples, this should include some physical touch, which will help your relationship and your anxiety levels.[2] Also make sure that the first thing you say to your loved one when you reunite at the end of the day is something positive rather than complaining, whining, or handing out honey do's (all easy traps to fall into!).

If you're single or you'd rather focus on your relationships with friends or other family members, you can ask yourself what sort of nurturing and encouragement these other people you have close relationships with need right now.

. . . .

The Learning Curve

At this point, you may be thinking that spotting your thinking errors and balancing your thinking is a heck of a lot of hard work and wondering if it will get easier. The good news is yes, it will. Spotting your thinking biases becomes more automatic the more you practice it. People tend to see rapid improvement in their anxiety symptoms when they first start correcting their thinking errors, but over time, you'll see a different type of improvement—one in which correcting anxiety-driven thinking errors becomes less and less of an effort.

For me personally, at this point it doesn't feel effortful *at all*. I still have the initial anxiety-driven thoughts, but now it's like they're spelling mistakes and I have a built-in autocorrect. Correcting anxiety-driven thoughts has become as instinctive as having the anxious thoughts in the first place. When you get to this point yourself, you'll find it's easier to take events and stress in stride, and you'll notice that you naturally feel more (not totally) mellow and chilled out. I'm still someone who likes to be prepared and be on the lookout for potential problems, but I now have plenty of moments of Zen too.

Through paying attention to your thinking errors and avoidance patterns on an ongoing basis, you can get to this point too. However, you don't always need to be on the lookout for thinking errors. Instead, go hunting for them only when you're feeling blue, anxious, overwhelmed, or stuck. When you get stuck or feel distressed, use that as a cue to ask yourself whether your top thinking errors are contributing.

After the Fact or At the Time

If you've been working on your thinking errors for only a few months so far, then you're probably still at the stage where you mostly notice the errors after the fact. Going forward, you'll find some situations in which you're able to spot a thinking error at or close to the time it occurs. For example, you might notice yourself feeling upset about something that has happened during the day and later that evening realize you've been mind reading: guessing what someone else thinks without knowing if it's actually the case.

Expect to have a mixture of these situations and those when you notice your thinking error only after you've been walking around buying into that sucker for months or even years. You might get some new information or evidence and only then realize you've been holding on to a distorted thought.

For example, I recently had a situation in which I was under the impression that a mentor was disappointed with what I had achieved in my career because I hadn't continued in the research field. Out of the blue, I got information that, in reality, the mentor was very impressed with what I'd achieved. The new information corrected that long-held example of mind reading. No matter how good you get at uncovering your thinking errors, sometimes you'll still get sucked in by them. Take comfort in the fact that the "Better late than never principle" applies! The more you zero in on which thinking errors are the most common causes of your anxious feelings, the more you'll be able to detect them on the fly.

The same strategies will also work for unsticking yourself from your most problematic behavioral traps. Just like with your thinking errors, use feeling anxious, stuck, or overwhelmed as your cue to ask yourself whether any of your most common behavioral traps are the culprit.

Make sure you have a plan for an alternative action you can take when you notice yourself sucked into your most frequent behavioral traps. For example, if you've set a goal so lofty you get frozen by feelings of being overwhelmed, then your alternative action would be revising that goal down to the point where you don't feel frozen anymore. Unstick yourself from your behavioral traps at the time when possible. Otherwise, add them to the agenda for your weekly check-in.

Managing Anxiety Doesn't Have to Be a Full-Time Job

If you're thinking that you don't want to spend your whole life managing your anxiety, then you are thinking on the right track. There are a few different approaches you can use for continuing to improve your Anxiety Toolkit skills without feeling like managing your anxiety is your second (or third) full-time job.

We've covered one approach—simplifying which thinking biases are your focus on a day-to-day basis and then doing a weekly check-in to address traps you didn't manage to successfully navigate at the time.

A second approach is to mark your calendar to come back and revisit all the material you've read in this book. If you put the book away, go live your life, and then revisit it six months later, you will come back as an intermediate-level cognitive behavioral self-scientist rather than as a beginner. You'll find that you relate to the material in different ways at that point because you already have a basic level of familiarity with the concepts.

A third approach is something that will appeal to people who enjoy thinking about their thinking, people who enjoy doing self-reflection. There are heaps of thinking errors that are common to virtually everyone and aren't necessarily associated with being anxiety-prone. If you're looking to further bump up your cognitive behavioral IQ, you might want to broaden your focus to detecting when and how you fall into those thinking traps. Should you choose to do this, I've put together an online cheat sheet of 50 common thinking errors (see TheAnxietyToolkit .com/resources).

Some people find that the idea of learning about more thinking biases is overwhelming at this stage of their learning. Other people like to shift away from focusing on anxiety, and find it comforting that thinking errors are normal and common to everyone. By learning about other common thinking biases, you can keep improving your understanding of cognitive behavioral psychology without focusing on anxiety all the time. Improving your ability to detect your thinking errors across the board will filter through to help you better detect your anxiety-related patterns.

In the next chapter, we'll do some advance troubleshooting of problems that sometimes get in the way of lowering anxiety. People don't usually realize that these issues are what's impeding their progress, which is why I'm going to point them out for you here.

CHAPTER 10

Areas Where People
Get Tripped Up

This chapter continues the theme of the prior chapter: You've got a well-stocked toolkit of skills for coping with your anxiety, and you're moving into the consolidation phase. Now, we'll shift our focus to common problems that might trip you up during this phase without you realizing what the issue is. When you can identify these problem areas, you'll be able to sidestep them and accelerate your progress toward a lower-anxiety life.

Take the following quiz to see how this chapter pertains to you. Choose the answer that *best* applies. If no answer is the perfect fit, pick whichever is the closest.

1. How's your lifestyle balance?

(A) I always have daily restorative time, even if it's just 10 minutes of not doing anything.

(B) I have some stress bottlenecks that could use some unclogging.

(C) I have so little lifestyle balance that even hearing the phrase stresses me out.

2. Are you still highly self-critical?

(A) Nope, I'm a self-compassion machine.

(B) I've improved in the self-compassion department, but sometimes I still act like a drill sergeant toward myself.

(C) I suspect I am still self-critical, but mostly I fail to notice I'm doing it.

3. How clear are you on the difference between ruminating/worrying and problem solving?

(A) Crystal.

(B) I am mostly clear on this. There are occasional times I mistake ruminating or worrying for problem solving.

(C) I still spend a lot of time thinking about problems in a way that doesn't really translate to effective action.

4. When you're experiencing stress or anxiety, do you put some boundaries on the extent to which you discuss those stressful topics or anxieties with others?

(A) I hit the sweet spot of talking about stressful situations or anxiety only to the extent that's useful.

(B) I don't choose times to talk about stressful topics as wisely as I could.

(C) Sometimes stress and anxiety are on my mind so much, I end up talking about them all the time.

5. **How much time and effort do you spend trying to change other people?**

(A) Only an amount that is useful.

(B) Probably a bit more than is useful.

(C) I repeatedly return to the same thoughts about how I'd like others to change. It's a futile exercise in frustration for everyone concerned, but I'm stuck in the trap of doing the same things and expecting different results.

6. **Does fear of panic attacks impede your enjoyment of life?**

(A) No.

(B) Not really, but I have some fear of how I'd cope if I had a panic attack.

(C) Yes, there are some experiences I opt out of for fear of having a panic attack.

Here's how to interpret your scores. If you scored:

Mostly A's

You're ahead of the game and aren't likely to get tripped up by some of the common pitfalls that affect other people and can cause anxiety to persist. But by reading this chapter, you're likely to gain a few insights into how you can optimize further.

Mostly B's

There are certain pitfalls that can cause anxiety to persist even when people are doing everything right in terms of using their toolkit of skills. Your answers indicate you're at risk of at least some of these. Reading this chapter will allow you to identify which pitfalls you may be vulnerable to and find solutions.

Mostly C's

You're at high risk of some stumbling blocks that can cause anxiety to persist, despite having done hard work on learning cognitive behavioral skills. Pay close attention to the information in this chapter in order to avoid these pitfalls and move from C's to A's.

The road to success isn't always smooth. You'll encounter rocks and potholes. But these challenges aren't insurmountable—you just need to navigate around them. The same goes for navigating a life with anxiety. There are common areas where people tend to get tripped up. Knowing what these pitfalls are will go a long way to helping you avoid them. If, as you read this chapter, you have a sense you're having a few too many "that's me" moments for comfort, remember I said that these are *common* pitfalls, so don't be too hard on yourself.

Lifestyle Imbalance

Many of the anxious people I've met are prone to excessive responsibility taking. They really don't like to let anyone down and typically work hard to avoid conflict or other people being potentially unhappy with them. And they usually have high standards for self-performance. What is all this a recipe for? Taking on too much.

Deep down, many people know what lifestyle changes they need to make to reduce their stress. It could be quitting a job that's never going to be just 40 hours a week because your boss continually pushes the boundaries to squeeze more and more work out of you. It might be having an awkward conversation in which other parties try to guilt-trip you into maintaining extra roles and responsibilities that you at some point agreed to take on. It could be challenging intolerance of uncertainty and giving up some control by outsourcing some tasks. Or, for a segment of anxiety-prone people, it could be learning to tolerate thoughts about being unworthy that you experience if you're not working all the time.

Everyone needs restorative time to process and recover from daily stress. As anxiety-prone people, we often need to build in this restorative time to process anxiety-provoking events and work up to doing things. If you have work/tasks squeezed too tightly into your life, then the natural anxiety that this triggers isn't a false alarm—it's a true alarm that's alerting you to the need to make a change.

Lifestyle changes often make a huge difference in the reserves and resources people have available to cope with stress. There is a limit to how effective internal changes are ever going to be if the root of the problem is your schedule. Time and time again I've observed the following pattern in my therapy clients: If their life is excessively busy, then reducing their schedule results in them finding it far easier to make better choices.

One barrier to making lifestyle changes is often social comparison. You cannot compare yourself to others when it comes to finding a schedule that works for you (well, you can, but it won't be helpful). A schedule that feels manageable and balanced for someone else might not be right for you.

Experiment: Changes in how you feel are going to come from making a mixture of external changes, like changes in how you spend your time, and internal changes, like working on your thinking. What are the psychological barriers you need to overcome to build more restorative time into your day?

Ongoing Self-Criticism

If there is any anxiety habit that seems particularly hard to break, it's self-criticism, but it's a habit that needs to be broken. When you use self-compassion rather than self-criticism to cope with stuff that doesn't go according to plan, you'll notice that you start making far better choices. Self-kindness creates mental space, where you can think more clearly about what problem needs to be solved, and will help give you confidence that you've got the goods to be able to solve your own problems.

Experiment: Dr. Kristin Neff, who is one of the leading experts on self-compassion, has generously made her self-compassion quiz available for anyone to take on her website.[1] Give this short quiz a try. The quiz will autoscore and let you know if you have room for improvement in the self-compassion department.

If your self-compassion score is low, put it on your calendar to retake the self-compassion quiz at intervals. You could choose monthly or three-month intervals. If you want to be nerdtastic, plot your scores on a graph and make sure they're headed in the positive direction.

Kristin's website (self-compassion.org) and her book *Self-Compassion* both include suggested exercises to increase self-compassion. The themes of some of these, such as mindfulness, will already be familiar to you from the work you've done here. If you need to improve your self-compassion, consider trying some of these exercises, plus the one I've included in Chapter 5. Self-compassion is a hot topic in psychology right now, so you can also search online for other exercises you may be interested in trying.

A heads-up: Self-compassion exercises may sound a little woo-woo or New Agey to some readers when you first encounter them. If an exercise you find doesn't appeal to you, search for others that are a better fit for your preferences.

Allowing Endless Information Seeking, Rumination, and Worry

The idea of allowing rumination or worry seems a bit silly at first. Who would want to have free-floating rumination or worry on an ongoing basis? However, remember that rumination and worry often masquerade as preparing to take action or preparing to solve a problem that might come up in the future.

People often allow themselves to endlessly think about how they might take action in the future; why they haven't taken action; why other people act the way they do; or a decision, a problem, or a possible problem. As we've covered, problem solving should generally involve concretely defining what the problem is, generating a short list of your best options for moving forward, picking something, and deciding when and where you're going to implement that solution.

If you're doing some other type of thinking but mentally labeling what you're doing as "problem solving" or "planning action," question whether it really is. Being in thinking-only mode for long periods is comforting in the same way that overeating junk food for long periods is. It feels comfortable in the moment, but in the long term, you end up far from where you wanted to be.

There's an element of art rather than science in figuring out the difference between useful thinking and not useful thinking. For example, some of my best ideas come from allowing my mind to drift back to work issues while I'm out walking and ostensibly taking a break from working. There are other times when allowing my mind to drift back to work feels more unhelpful—for example, mentally running over choices or conversations while I'm driving home in the car.

Experiment: For you, when is letting your mind wander generally productive? When isn't it? Identify at least one example of each.

The Self-Improvement Addicts Club

This next point won't be applicable to everyone, but it's worth mentioning for the segment of people for whom this does affect.

If you're someone who constantly reads self-improvement information, you might want to set some boundaries for yourself. Reading new self-improvement materials can become a crutch for some people. That is, you're always trying to find the magic missing piece of information that will solve your self-puzzle and make action taking seem easier and more certain than it's ever going to be. You need to make sure you're translating your most important insights into action rather than just doing more reading.

Experiment: If you're a card-carrying member of the all-reading, no-action self-improvement-addicts club, try taking a break from reading new self-improvement material. For example, you might decide, "I'm not going to read any new self-improvement information for a couple of weeks" and see how that goes.

The issue isn't so much about trying new types of self-improvement; it's about continually reading to gain insights without taking much action or without prioritizing the most important insights you need to apply. In the two weeks you're taking off from reading new information, commit to applying one behavioral strategy in your life that you've previously read about. Choose that strategy now by first generating a list of three to six options and then picking one of those options. Plan when and where you're going to implement the strategy you've chosen.

Talking About Stress or Anxiety All the Time

If you're experiencing a stressful life event that involves ongoing conversations with others, try putting some limits on when you have those conversations. This advice especially applies to times like when you're planning a wedding. Here's another example: A client of mine had a legal action pending, and the issues surrounding it were also affecting many of her neighbors. She spent a ton of time keeping up with what was going on with the neighbors who were in a similar situation and discussing any information she'd heard or read with her husband. The problem was that it was making her miserable. In reality, she didn't need to be doing so much ongoing monitoring of the local and neighborhood news. Her lawyer was communicating regularly with her about where things were at, and making requests for additional information as needed. Doing endless mental preparation to deal with potential (aka might-never-eventuate) problems meant that she was not trusting her ability to make appropriate judgments when needed. In my client's case, dealing with issues as they arose was something she was very capable of doing.

Putting boundaries on when you talk about stressful plans

and situations with other people can be as simple as waiting until the end of the day to convey updates to each other rather than sending texts or emails during the day. In some cases, having a designated meeting with your spouse or partner once a week to discuss a particular topic works better than talking about it daily.

It's also good to limit the extent to which you talk about how anxious you feel; don't give out a daily anxiety update like a weather update. Friends and loved ones sometimes tire of constant anxiety updates and rundowns on all the things that are stressing you out.

Experiment: What boundaries do you need to put around how much you talk about a particular topic with other people?

Taking Too Much Responsibility for Other People

Coming back to the theme of excessive responsibility taking: Anxious people sometimes spend too much time and energy trying to change other people. Be aware if you're doing this as a way of avoiding focusing on yourself and your own goals. Of course it's easier to shift focus to what others could change rather than deal with the psychological work that's sitting on your own plate. Another factor that can contribute to anxiety-prone people getting caught in this trap is their tendency to overpersist with actions beyond the point of what's useful. You try and try and try in situations where giving up might be a better choice.

Experiment: Is there someone you are trying to change and it's not working? Are you caught in the pattern of trying the same things and expecting different results? What would giving up on trying to change that other person look like? For example, in a situation where you'd normally complain to the person about his or her behavior, what could you do instead?

Fear of Panic Attacks

First of all, if you haven't had panic attacks before, there is no reason to think you'll start having them now. The following tips are for people who've had the odd panic attack in the past and would like to feel better equipped for how to handle them.

Panic attacks are short and sharp and tend to reach peak intensity within 10 to 20 minutes (although some symptoms may persist for an hour or more).[2] Our bodies are designed for these extreme anxiety responses to last only a short period of time. There is no one in the history of the planet whose anxiety system has ever become stuck in panic attack mode permanently. It's a physiological impossibility. We have one part of our nervous system that boots up the panic response and another part that shuts that response down. What goes up must come down.

You actually don't need to do anything to stop a panic attack. You could do anything, do nothing, or do completely the wrong thing and the panic attack would stop on its own. The suggestions in this section will help you feel more prepared, but if you forget them all and happen to have a panic attack at a time when you don't have access to this book, you will still be absolutely fine. Take comfort in the fact that your body knows what to do to reset itself after the panic response is triggered.

If you ever find yourself feeling like a panicky, exploding fireball of anxiety, then your first go-to strategies should be physiological. Forget focusing on your thinking errors. When you're really worked up in panicky mode, give yourself a break from trying to dig around in your thoughts. By evolutionary design, you're in reaction mode when you're panicking, not contemplation mode. Your anxiety system has wound itself up to its emergency fight, flight, or freeze mode, and you want to dial that back. Here are some strategies to try:

- **Slow breathing.** You're going to need to have practiced this for it to feel comfortable when you feel panicky. See Chapter 4 for advice on how to practice.

- **Physical touch.** Get some oxytocin release happening by rubbing/stroking your arm (the skin, not through your clothes) or getting a long hug from someone.

- **Temperature.** A great way to disrupt your nervous system and feel physically calmer (which will slow and calm your thoughts) is to change your temperature. You can go hot or icy. Choose what works for you. For example, heat might be a bath or shower. Ice could involve breaking up some ice cubes and sucking the ice chips.

A more extreme version of the ice technique involves putting your face into a basin of ice water (tap water + some ice). This technique comes from dialectical behavioral therapy (DBT), a therapy developed by Dr. Marsha Linehan.[3] If you want to use the face-in-ice-water technique, do an Internet search for

"DBT dive reflex," and you'll find different versions of the instructions and some variations you can try. The technique is designed to stimulate the effect that happens if you were submerged in cold water and your body needed to conserve energy. In this scenario, one of the things your body naturally does is to turn down the volume on systems that use up a lot of energy, such as . . . you guessed it, the anxiety system.

Note that the dive reflex technique is not recommended for people with any history or risk of heart problems or for people with eating disorders who may have heart vulnerabilities due to their eating disorder. *Don't just use my brief description here; look up some more detailed instructions and warnings, and consult your physician before trying this.* If you don't have ice, try getting something cold out of your freezer and putting it on your face for a few seconds, then repeating. Wrap the frozen item in a thin layer of cloth, like an old T-shirt or a thin towel.

- **DBT distress tolerance skills.**[4] There are some other great techniques for dealing with extreme anxiety that also come from dialectical behavioral therapy. DBT is a cousin of cognitive behavioral therapy in that there are some similarities and some differences between the two approaches. DBT was originally designed as a therapy for people who have borderline personality disorder, which involves, among other things, feeling emotions very intensely. Therefore, if you do an Internet search for "DBT distress tolerance," you will find numerous suggestions that can help when you're feeling very extreme emotions.

- **Activity.** Burning off some excess energy usually helps you feel calmer if you're feeling very distressed; try jumping on your kids' trampoline, for example.

- **The milk, milk, milk technique.**[5] This technique was first described 100 years ago, but it's been popularized as part of another type of therapy called acceptance and commitment therapy, or ACT as it's often called (as in the word *act*, not A.C.T.). This therapy was first developed by Dr. Steven Hayes and has since been extensively studied.[6] Like dialectical behavioral therapy, ACT can also be considered a cousin of cognitive behavioral therapy. There are important differences between the two approaches as well as important similarities.

  Milk, milk, milk involves taking a trigger word from whatever repetitive thought you're having—such as *breakup, alone, overwhelmed, foolish*—and repeating that word as fast as possible for 30 seconds to two minutes. The technique is called milk, milk, milk because when people practice it with a therapist, the practice word used is *milk*.

  How does the technique work? When you expose yourself over and over to whatever word is triggering your distress, it starts to lose its power in triggering painful memories and becomes just a sound.

- **Find company.** If you have a panic attack and you've never had one before, you might want to ask someone to hang out with you—by phone, on Skype, or in person—while the panic attack is working itself out. You'll get through a panic attack alone, but if it's the first time you've had one, you'll likely feel more comfortable if you have someone with you. Try not to have this be someone like an ex-boyfriend or ex-girlfriend, where reopening that can of worms could complicate things later.

A final note about panic attacks: Having one or several panic attacks doesn't mean you're going to have them all the time. I know plenty of people who are prone to getting a panic attack once every 5 to 10 years or so. It's unpleasant, but by far the most unpleasant aspect is the fear of having another one. Notice that I labeled this section "*fear* of panic attacks." It's much more common for fear of future panic attacks to be the thing that traps people in ongoing anxiety than the problem being the actual panic attacks.

If you happen to have panic disorder, meaning you get frequent panic attacks, then rest assured that getting panic disorder treatment from a cognitive behavioral therapist who is using a program specifically designed to treat panic attacks has a very high success rate. Your therapy should include something called *interoceptive exposure* because panic disorder treatments that include this are the most effective.[7] You can try a self-help version of interoceptive exposure online as part of a free program.[8]

If your panic attack has something to do with drugs or alcohol then you should seek professional help as your judgment will be impaired and a drug-fueled panic attack is more unpredictable than a regular one.

CHAPTER 11

Liking Your Natural Self vs. Tolerating Your Natural Self

Moving from tolerating your nature to liking yourself is our final step. You've done a great job making it to the final chapter.

Take the following quiz to see how this chapter pertains to you. Choose the answer that *best* applies. If no answer is the perfect fit, pick whichever is the closest.

1. How "in like" are you with your core self?

(A) I feel a sense of peace and contentment with who I am.

(B) Some days I think I'm an OK person, but it's very up and down.

(C) I regularly wrestle with a sense of disliking my nature.

2. How easy is it for you to recognize ways in which you're *not* a particularly anxiety-prone person?

(A) Although I'm anxiety-prone, I also recognize situations in which I'm confident and self-assured.

(B) I tend to mostly pay attention to situations in which I'm anxious and overlook situations in which I'm not.

(C) My self-identity is that I'm virtually never confident, self-assured, or optimistic.

3. Are you clear about what your strengths as a person are?

(A) I could rattle off a list right now.

(B) Mmm, sorta. I could name one or two character strengths, but I'd get stuck after that.

(C) I spend so much time thinking about my weaknesses, I haven't thought about my strengths.

4. Do you still have lurking fixed mindsets—beliefs that you can't improve skills you see as critical to your ultimate success?

(A) Nope, I'm good to go.

(B) I still underestimate my ability to approach certain skills in ways that utilize my strengths and talents.

(C) There are still things I see as essential skills for success that I believe I can't be good at.

5. Do you have people in your support network who encourage you to be self-accepting and help you feel positive about your nature?

(A) Yes.

(B) One or two people, but I wish I had more.

(C) No.

6. **Do you have people in your support network who encourage you to take action when you're feeling hesitant?**

(A) Yes.

(B) Maybe one.

(C) No.

Here's how to interpret your scores. If you scored:

Mostly A's

You're well on your way to being self-accepting and confident in yourself as a person. You have people in your network who help you see your strengths. You're able to see your nature as having some fluidity; for example, you can see that you're sometimes confident and sometimes anxious, rather than seeing yourself in all-or-nothing terms.

Mostly B's

You're on the bubble in terms of whether you generally feel positive about your nature. Your sense of a positive self probably goes up and down with your mood and things that are happening in your life. This chapter will help you develop your capacity to see your core strengths clearly.

Mostly C's

Your negative view of yourself is still a significant challenge that gets in the way of having lower anxiety. You probably have some more serious types of negative character beliefs, like "I'm incompetent," "I'm unworthy," or "I'm weak." This chapter will help you strengthen alternative beliefs.

When clients have finished their regular therapy sessions, they're usually at a stage of being more tolerant and accepting of their anxiety-proneness. They're successfully working with their anxious nature more productively and without as much emotional drama. However, they often still feel like their anxiety-proneness is a burden or weakness. Saying they were "in like" with their fundamental nature would be a bit of a stretch.

It's really important that you like who you are. Provided you're not a serial killer, no one deserves the emotional pain of going through life not liking themselves (yes you, even if you have flaws). This chapter provides directions for how you can continue your journey toward actually liking, rather than begrudgingly tolerating, your natural self.

Notice When You Don't React to Situations in an Anxious Way

Even the most anxiety-prone person doesn't always react to situations in an anxious way. Start paying attention to situations in which you:

- Naturally make positive predictions
- Feel confident in your ability to complete challenging tasks
- Receive feedback without personalizing it or catastrophizing
- Ask for what you want without being excessively hesitant
- Feel accepting and relaxed

Start to notice how you are sometimes anxiety-prone and sometimes confident, rather than thinking about anxiety-proneness and confidence as being mutually exclusive traits. Without exception, all the clients I've seen for anxiety have areas of their life where they're naturally confident and self-assured. Many of them appear confident. It's not fake or false—their anxiety and their confidence exist together as parts of their personality. In fact, people often compliment me on being a very confident person. As you know from reading my examples, I'm also very anxiety-prone. For me, neither "I'm confident" nor "I'm anxiety-prone" is more true than the other. They both exist together as part of my nature. I'm sure the same is true for you. If you doubt it, remember *The Wizard of Oz,* in which the Lion worried he didn't have bravery and the Tin Man worried he didn't have a heart. They had those things all along; they just didn't recognize those qualities in themselves.

Why am I making the point that even the most anxiety-prone people aren't anxious all the time? Noticing the grayness and fuzziness involved in defining yourself in any one particular way will help your ongoing development of flexible thinking. The purpose of seeing the grayness of your nature is to not label yourself too rigidly.

Experiment: What's a recent example of a situation that someone might've found anxiety provoking, but you didn't?

Know Your Character Strengths

Try identifying your top five strengths as a person. Don't just think about the work domain. Remember I said "as a person," not "as a worker bee." If these don't spring to mind immediately, start paying attention to when you do a good job on something or you feel good about yourself, and ask yourself which strengths are contributing to those situations.

If you want to take a formal strengths test, you can search online and try some out. There are plenty that are available free online. Sometimes the ones that have the most science behind them aren't always the ones that people report finding the most helpful or interesting.

Once you have a short list of your top five strengths, try referring to this list when you have a problem you need to overcome. For example, if your strength is resourcefulness, then remember this strength when you need to solve a problem. To increase your psychological flexibility, try applying your strengths in new ways compared to how you'd usually apply them.[1] For example, if you'd usually apply your resourcefulness to figuring out how to do a task yourself, try using your resourcefulness to find someone you could outsource that work to. If you'd usually apply your strength of conscientiousness to doing a task extremely thoroughly, try applying your conscientiousness to limiting the amount of time and energy you invest in the task and sticking to that limit.

Experiment: List your top five strengths as a person. Since you're free to revise your list at any point (it's yours after all), don't get too perfectionistic about it. Once you have your list, identify a task you currently need to do. How could you apply one of your top five strengths to approach that task in a new way?

Challenge Remaining Fixed Mindsets

An area where people usually have ongoing work to do is fixed mindsets—the belief that your capacities are fixed and can't be changed—which, as we've discussed, tends to lead to under-achievement.

Keep hunting down your fixed mindsets. Why is this so important? Fixed mindsets can leave people with a sense that something is holding them back or that they're deficient in some way. Back in Chapter 6, we dealt with the fixed mindset "I'm not an ideas person." A couple of other fixed mindsets that commonly come up are "I'm no good at networking" or "I'm no good at negotiating" (an example I briefly mentioned in Chapter 4).

The key to overcoming a fixed mindset is finding a way of practicing the "fixed" skill that's both effective and a good fit for you. Consider networking as an example. I like to network through professional Facebook groups. Participants use the groups to ask and answer questions and share useful tidbits of information. The beauty of these groups is that people can dip in and out of participating when they have the time and inclination. By finding ways to practice networking that suit my strengths (using technology) and preferences (don't involve dressing up), I've changed my fixed mindset about being bad at networking and being unable to improve. It's even changed my belief that I dislike networking.

Whenever you find yourself still clinging on to a fixed mindset, ask yourself how you could practice that skill in a way that suits your nature, talents, and preferences. If you're feeling bad about yourself, ask yourself if a fixed mindset could be the issue and what a growth mindset alternative would be.

Experiment: When little kids say "I don't like math," usually their underlying issue is that they find math hard. What's a skill you dislike (like networking or negotiating)? Skills you dislike are often a fertile hunting ground for fixed mindsets that are still hiding and could possibly be challenged. What are some ways you could potentially pursue the disliked skill that would utilize your core strengths and interests? You don't have to commit to doing anything; this is just a thought exercise. For example, someone who is into chemistry but not into cooking could start thinking about the chemistry aspects of cooking.

Replace Negative Character Labels

Negative character labels are an even more serious problem than fixed mindsets. Examples of negative character labels include "I'm selfish," "I'm needy," "I'm unlovable," "I'm weak," "I'm defective," "I'm incompetent," and "I'm worthless." Such an uplifting list! Those negative beliefs sound quite dramatic when written down on the page, and sometimes people don't realize that they hold those beliefs about themselves. If your immediate reaction is to say, "Oh, I don't think any of those things about myself" or "Only someone who was super depressed would think those things," then take an extra second to make sure you're not even partially buying into these types of thoughts about yourself. It might be that you believe a negative character label only 20% of the time, but even that can still be an issue.

There are two types of negative character labels. Both can be changed. One type is very stable. For example, you believe you are incompetent, and you have never believed anything else, not even when you are in a positive mood. The other type is the type that goes up and down with your mood, anxiety, and stress. When your mood is low, you believe the negative character label much more strongly than when your mood is positive. If your negative character label changes due to transient things like your mood, anxiety, or stress, this can help you start to see that the belief is a product of these things rather than true.

Experiment: To replace negative character labels, try the following steps:

1. Pick a new, positive character label that you would prefer. For example, if your old belief is "I'm incompetent," you would likely pick "I'm competent."

2. Rate how much you currently believe the old negative character label on a scale of 0 (= I don't believe it at all) to 100

(= I believe it completely). Do the same for the new positive belief. For example, you might say you believe "I'm incompetent" at level 95 and believe "I'm competent" at level 10 (the numbers don't need to add up to 100).

3. Create a Positive Data Log and a Historical Data Log. Strengthening your new, positive character label is often a more helpful approach than attempting to hack away at the old, negative one. I'm going to give you two experiments that will help do this.

Positive Data Log. For two weeks, commit to writing down evidence that supports your new, positive character belief. For example, if you are trying to boost your belief in the thought "I'm competent" and you show up to an appointment on time, you can write that down as evidence.

Don't fall into the cognitive trap of discounting some of the evidence. For example, if you make a mistake and then sort it out, it's evidence of competence, not incompetence, so you could put that in your Positive Data Log.

Historical Data Log. This log looks back at periods of your life and finds evidence from those time periods that supports your positive character belief. This experiment helps people believe that the positive character quality represents part of their enduring nature. To do this experiment, split your life into whatever size chunks you want to split it into, such as four- to six-year periods. If you're only in your 20s, then you might choose three- or four-year periods.

To continue the prior example, if you're working on the belief "I'm competent," then evidence from childhood might be things like learning to walk, talk, or make friends. You figured these things out. From your teen years, your evidence of general competency at life might be getting your driver's license (yes, on the third try still counts). Evidence from your early college years could be things like successfully choosing a major and passing your courses. Evidence for after you finished your formal education might be related to finding work to support yourself and finding housing. You should include evidence in the social domain, like finding someone you wanted to date or figuring out how to break up with someone when you realized that relationship wasn't the right fit for you. The general idea is to prove to yourself that "I'm competent" is more true than "I'm incompetent."

Other positive character beliefs you might try to strengthen could be things like "I'm strong" (not weak), "I'm worthy of love" (not unlovable), and "I'm worthy of respect" (not worthless). Sometimes the flipside of a negative character belief is obvious, as in the case of strong/weak, but sometimes there are a couple of possible options that could be considered opposites; in this case, you can choose.

4. Rerate how much you believe the negative and positive character labels. There should have been a little bit of change as a result of doing the data logs. For example, you might now believe "I'm incompetent" at only 50 instead

of 95, and believe "I'm competent" at 60 instead of 10. You've probably had your negative character belief for a long time, so changing it isn't like making a pack of instant noodles.

If you want to do further work in this area, some of my clients have enjoyed a book called *Reinventing Your Life*.[2] It's a resource you can use to shift your negative character labels if you think that's something you need to work on. You could also see a cognitive behavioral therapist and let him or her know that you've done some work on thinking errors like mind reading, personalizing, and negative predictions but that you'd like to do some work on core beliefs. *Core beliefs* is the common clinical term for what I've called positive and negative character labels.

Note: The Positive Data Log and Historical Data Log exercises are based on exercises developed by Dr. Christine Padesky.[3]

Find Your Support Network

Most of this book has been focused on helping you work on your internal world. I want to use this last section to get you thinking about the roles other people could play, and perhaps have played, in (1) helping you like and accept your nature and (2) encouraging you to do things that are meaningful to you but that make you feel vulnerable.

People who are anxious tend to benefit from having people in their support network who provide the following functions:

- **An accepter.** Someone who you feel 100% accepted by, who helps you be more self-accepting. This person helps you see that your imperfections and quirky temperament aren't fatal flaws that are going to result in being rejected by others. While accepting of your nature, this person should be someone who sets some limits, such as not playing into it when you've whipped yourself into a worry frenzy.

- **A nudger.** Someone who encourages you to go for it. Ideally this should be someone who has already experienced success in the field where you want success and who gives you the little push you need to attempt to follow in their footsteps. If you've already achieved a level of success, this person will be someone who is a step or two ahead of you.

- **A clear thinker.** Someone who you can talk to about decisions you're contemplating and who will say something sensible. They won't solve your problems for you, but the person will be a sounding board who will chip in with useful comments, which will help you move your thinking forward.

You won't be able to make these support people magically appear out of thin air. Over time, build, nurture, and treasure relationships with people who can provide one or more of these functions. Research on relationships has shown that our support people help us see positive qualities in ourselves that we fail to see in ourselves.[4] The right kinds of support people can help you appreciate your multidimensional nature more clearly and help you break free of the excessively narrow or negative ways in which you might see yourself. As your self-confidence, self-knowledge, and self-acceptance bloom, you'll find it easier and easier to take action, even when those actions provoke a sense of anxiety and vulnerability.

CONCLUSION

. . . .

This is the end of our journey together for now. Thank you for the hard work you've put into understanding and learning how to navigate your anxiety. Over the coming months, you'll no doubt have lots of opportunities to apply the insights you've learned here to your life. Through that process, the insights you've gained will turn into skills, which you will then always have at your disposal to cope with any situation.

Very best wishes,
Alice

ACKNOWLEDGMENTS

Much of this book is based on my training in cognitive behavioral models of anxiety and CBT. My thanks go to all the thousands of researchers who have contributed to our collective understanding of the psychology of anxiety. I'd also like to thank my clients, who, through their willingness to work hard and collaboratively, have taught me as much about the psychology of individuals as I have taught them.

Numerous other people have been involved in bringing this book to life. My super agent, Giles Anderson, was influential in the genesis of this book and helped me go from book idea to book contract in just a few months. My editor at Perigee Books, Meg Leder, has been just the type of editor any author would hope for—she has made this book better.

I've been lucky to have some wonderful mentors throughout my psychology career; Professor Garth Fletcher, Dr. Fran Vertue, and Professor Janet Latner have given me both skills and confidence.

For reading countless drafts and reminding me when I'm not taking my own advice, I'd like to thank my spouse, Dr. Kathryn Burnell. Of course it's a bit sappy to mention my mom, but to my mom—I love you, and knowing you are always there for me is what has given me the underlying feelings of safety and security that have allowed me to pursue my goals.

Writing a book can be quite a solitary process and might have felt lonely had it not been for the wonderful community of other psychology writers I have met through blogging at PsychologyToday.com. My fellow blogger-authors have been very generous with their friendship and advice, including Dr. Guy Winch; Toni Bernhard, JD; Professor Art Markman; Dr. Susan Newman; Dr. Mindy Greenstein; Dr. Barb Markway; Lynne Soraya; and Meg Selig.

REFERENCES

Aldao, Amelia, Susan Nolen-Hoeksema, and Susanne Schweizer. "Emotion-Regulation Strategies across Psychopathology: A Meta-Analytic Review." *Clinical Psychology Review* 30, no. 2 (2010): 217–37.

Allen, David. *Getting Things Done: The Art of Stress-Free Productivity.* New York: Penguin, 2002.

Arch, Joanna J., Georg H. Eifert, Carolyn Davies, Jennifer C. Plumb Vilardaga, Raphael D. Rose, and Michelle G. Craske. "Randomized Clinical Trial of Cognitive Behavioral Therapy (CBT) Versus Acceptance and Commitment Therapy (ACT) for Mixed Anxiety Disorders." *Journal of Consulting and Clinical Psychology* 80, no. 5 (2012): 750.

Aron, Elaine N. *The Highly Sensitive Person.* New York: Broadway Books, 1997.

Aron, Elaine N., and Arthur Aron. "Sensory-Processing Sensitivity and Its Relation to Introversion and Emotionality." *Journal of Personality and Social Psychology* 73, no. 2 (1997): 345.

Barrett, Paula M., Ronald M. Rapee, Mark M. Dadds, and Sharon M. Ryan. "Family Enhancement of Cognitive Style in Anxious and Aggressive Children." *Journal of Abnormal Child Psychology* 24, no. 2 (1996): 187–203.

Baumeister, Roy F., Arlene M. Stillwell, and Todd F. Heatherton. "Guilt: An Interpersonal Approach." *Psychological Bulletin* 115, no. 2 (1994): 243.

Beck, Judith S. *Cognitive Behavior Therapy: Basics and Beyond.* New York: Guilford Press, 2011.

Bernhard, Toni. "4 Tips for Slowing Down to Reduce Stress." *Psychology Today*, September 13, 2011. psychologytoday.com/blog/turning-straw-gold/201109/4-tips-slowing-down-reduce-stress.

"Big Five Personality Traits." Wikipedia. en.wikipedia.org/wiki/Big_Five_personality_traits.

Boyes, Alice. "5 Meditation Tips for Beginners." *Psychology Today*, March 18, 2013. psychologytoday.com/blog/in-practice/201303/5-meditation-tips-beginners.

Boyes, Alice. "7 Ways You Can Benefit from Procrastinating." *Psychology Today*, June 19, 2014. psychologytoday.com/blog/in-practice/201406/7-ways-you-can-benefit-procrastinating.

Boyes, Alice D., and Garth J. O. Fletcher. "Metaperceptions of Bias in Intimate Relationships." *Journal of Personality and Social Psychology* 92, no. 2 (2007): 286.

Breines, Juliana G., and Serena Chen. "Self-Compassion Increases Self-Improvement Motivation." *Personality and Social Psychology Bulletin* 38, no. 9 (2012): 1133–43.

Brown, Brené. "Listening to Shame." TED Talks, March 2012. ted.com/talks/brene_brown_listening_to_shame?language=en.

Butler, Andrew C., Jason E. Chapman, Evan M. Forman, and Aaron T. Beck. "The Empirical Status of Cognitive-Behavioral Therapy: A Review of Meta-Analyses." *Clinical Psychology Review* 26, no. 1 (2006): 17–31.

"Coping with Physical Alarms: Exposure—Part 1." Centre for Clinical Interventions. www.cci.health.wa.gov.au/docs/Panic-09_Exposure-1.pdf.

Derrick, Jaye L. "Energized by Television: Familiar Fictional Worlds Restore Self-Control." *Social Psychological and Personality Science* 4, no. 3 (2013): 299–307.

Dugas, Michel J., Patrick Gosselin, and Robert Ladouceur. "Intolerance of Uncertainty and Worry: Investigating Specificity in a Nonclinical Sample." *Cognitive Therapy and Research* 25, no. 5 (2001): 551–58.

Dweck, Carol. *Mindset: The New Psychology of Success*. New York: Random House, 2006.

Edwards, Susan L., Ronald M. Rapee, and John Franklin. "Postevent Rumination and Recall Bias for a Social Performance Event in High and Low Socially Anxious Individuals." *Cognitive Therapy and Research* 27, no. 6 (2003): 603–17.

References

Egan, Sarah J., Tracey D. Wade, and Roz Shafran. "Perfectionism as a Trans-diagnostic Process: A Clinical Review." *Clinical Psychology Review* 31, no. 2 (2011): 203–12.

Elliott, Elaine S., and Carol S. Dweck. "Goals: An Approach to Motivation and Achievement." *Journal of Personality and Social Psychology* 54, no. 1 (1988): 5.

"Facts & Statistics." Anxiety and Depression Association of America. adaa.org/about-adaa/press-room/facts-statistics.

Feske, Ulrike, and Dianne L. Chambless. "Cognitive Behavioral Versus Exposure Only Treatment for Social Phobia: A Meta-Analysis." *Behavior Therapy* 26, no. 4 (1995): 695–720.

Fry, Prem S., and Dominique L. Debats. "Perfectionism and the Five-Factor Personality Traits as Predictors of Mortality in Older Adults." *Journal of Health Psychology* 14, no. 4 (2009): 513–24.

"The Fundamental Attribution Error." Wikipedia. en.wikipedia.org/wiki/Fundamental_attribution_error.

Glenn, Daniel, Daniela Golinelli, Raphael D. Rose, Peter Roy-Byrne, Murray B. Stein, Greer Sullivan, Alexander Bystritsky, Cathy Sherbourne, and Michelle G. Craske. "Who Gets the Most out of Cognitive Behavioral Therapy for Anxiety Disorders? The Role of Treatment Dose and Patient Engagement." *Journal of Consulting and Clinical Psychology* 81, no. 4 (2013): 639.

Gollwitzer, Peter M., and Veronika Brandstätter. "Implementation Intentions and Effective Goal Pursuit." *Journal of Personality and Social Psychology* 73, no. 1 (1997): 186.

Gottman, John Mordechai, and Nan Silver. *The Seven Principles for Making Marriage Work*. New York: Random House, 1999.

Gould, Robert A., Michael W. Ott, and Mark H. Pollack. "A Meta-Analysis of Treatment Outcome for Panic Disorder." *Clinical Psychology Review* 15, no. 8 (1995): 819–44.

Halvorson, Heidi Grant, and E. Tory Higgins. *Focus: Use Different Ways of Seeing the World for Success and Influence*. New York: Plume, 2014.

Harvey, Allison G. "A Cognitive Model of Insomnia." *Behaviour Research and Therapy* 40, no. 8 (2002): 869–93.

Hofmann, Stefan G., Alice T. Sawyer, Ashley A. Witt, and Diana Oh. "The Effect of Mindfulness-Based Therapy on Anxiety and Depression: A Meta-Analytic Review." *Journal of Consulting and Clinical Psychology* 78, no. 2 (2010): 169.

Hofmann, Stefan G., and Jasper A. J. Smits. "Cognitive-Behavioral Therapy for Adult Anxiety Disorders: A Meta-Analysis of Randomized Placebo-Controlled Trials." *Journal of Clinical Psychiatry* 69, no. 4 (2008): 621.

Holahan, Charles J., Rudolf H. Moos, Carole K. Holahan, Penny L. Brennan, and Kathleen K. Schutte. "Stress Generation, Avoidance Coping, and Depressive Symptoms: A 10-Year Model." *Journal of Consulting and Clinical Psychology* 73, no. 4 (2005): 658.

Holt-Lunstad, Julianne, Wendy A. Birmingham, and Kathleen C. Light. "Influence of a 'Warm Touch' Support Enhancement Intervention Among Married Couples on Ambulatory Blood Pressure, Oxytocin, Alpha Amylase, and Cortisol." *Psychosomatic Medicine* 70, no. 9 (2008): 976–85.

"Intermittent Reinforcement." Out of the FOG. outofthefog.net/Common NonBehaviors/IntermittentReinforcement.html.

Iyengar, Sheena S., and Mark R. Lepper. "When Choice Is Demotivating: Can One Desire Too Much of a Good Thing?" *Journal of Personality and Social Psychology* 79, no. 6 (2000): 995.

Kotov, Roman, Wakiza Gamez, Frank Schmidt, and David Watson. "Linking 'Big' Personality Traits to Anxiety, Depressive, and Substance Use Disorders: A Meta-Analysis." *Psychological Bulletin* 136, no. 5 (2010): 768.

Kramer, Adam D. I., Jamie E. Guillory, and Jeffrey T. Hancock. "Experimental Evidence of Massive-Scale Emotional Contagion through Social Networks." *Proceedings of the National Academy of Sciences U.S.A.* 11, no. 24 (2014): 8788–90.

Leith, Karen P., and Roy F. Baumeister. "Empathy, Shame, Guilt, and Narratives of Interpersonal Conflicts: Guilt-Prone People Are Better at Perspective Taking." *Journal of Personality* 66, no. 1 (1998): 1–37.

Linehan, Marsha M. *Skills Training Manual for Treating Borderline Personality Disorder.* New York: Guilford Press, 1993.

Linehan, Marsha M., Martin Bohus, and Thomas R. Lynch. "Dialectical Behavior Therapy for Pervasive Emotion Dysregulation." In *Handbook of Emotion Regulation*, edited by James J. Gross. NewYork: Guilford Press, 2007.

Lyubomirsky, Sonja, Fazilet Kasri, Olivia Chang, and Irene Chung. "Ruminative Response Styles and Delay of Seeking Diagnosis for Breast Cancer Symptoms." *Journal of Social and Clinical Psychology* 25, no. 3 (2006): 276–304.

Markman, Art. "Changing Habits Beautifully." YouBeauty.com, August 16, 2011. youbeauty.com/mind/columns/a-beautiful-mind/changing-habits -beautifully.

Markman, Art. *Smart Thinking: Three Essential Keys to Solve Problems, Innovate, and Get Things Done.* New York: Perigee, 2012.

Markman, Art. "The Upside and Downside of Being Nice at Work." *Huffington Post*, March 30, 2012. huffingtonpost.com/art-markman-phd/ nice-people_b_1223492.html.

Masuda, Akihiko, Steven C. Hayes, Casey F. Sackett, and Michael P. Twohig. "Cognitive Defusion and Self-Relevant Negative Thoughts: Examining the Impact of a Ninety Year Old Technique." *Behaviour Research and Therapy* 42, no. 4 (2004): 477–85.

Mayer, John D., Laura J. McCormick, and Sara E. Strong. "Mood-Congruent Memory and Natural Mood: New Evidence." *Personality and Social Psychology Bulletin* 21 (1995): 736–36.

McGonigal, Kelly. "Does Self-Compassion or Criticism Motivate Self-Improvement?" *Psychology Today*, June 4, 2012. psychologytoday.com/ blog/the-science-willpower/201206/does-self-compassion-or-criticism -motivate-self-improvement.

McGonigal, Kelly. "How to Make Stress Your Friend." TED Talks, June

2013. ted.com/talks/kelly_mcgonigal_how_to_make_stress_your_ friend.

McKay, Matthew, Patrick Fanning, and Patricia Zurita Ona. *Mind and Emotions: A Universal Treatment for Emotional Disorders*. Oakland, CA: New Harbinger, 2011.

Murray, Sandra L., John G. Holmes, and Dale W. Griffin. "The Self-Fulfilling Nature of Positive Illusions in Romantic Relationships: Love Is Not Blind, but Prescient." *Journal of Personality and Social Psychology* 71, no. 6 (1996): 1155.

"Need for Cognition." Wikipedia. en.wikipedia.org/wiki/Need_for_ cognition.

Neff, Kristin. *Self-Compassion: Stop Beating Yourself Up and Leave Insecurity Behind*. New York: HarperCollins, 2011.

Neff, Kristin. "Test How Self-Compassionate You Are." Self-Compassion, 2009. self-compassion.org/test-your-self-compassion-level.html.

Norem, Julie K., and Edward C. Chang. "The Positive Psychology of Negative Thinking." *Journal of Clinical Psychology* 58, no. 9 (2002): 993–1001.

Olatunji, Bunmi O., Josh M. Cisler, and Brett J. Deacon. "Efficacy of Cognitive Behavioral Therapy for Anxiety Disorders: A Review of Meta-Analytic Findings." *Psychiatric Clinics of North America* 33, no. 3 (2010): 557–77.

Padesky, Christine A. "Schema Change Processes in Cognitive Therapy." *Clinical Psychology & Psychotherapy* 1, no. 5 (1994): 267–78.

"Panic Stations." Centre for Clinical Intervention. www.cci.health.wa.gov .au/resources/infopax.cfm?Info_ID=44.

Rapee, Ronald M., and Lina Lim. "Discrepancy Between Self- and Observer Ratings of Performance in Social Phobics." *Journal of Abnormal Psychology* 101, no. 4 (1992): 728.

Rashid, Tayyab, and Afroze Anjum. "340 Ways to Use VIA Character Strengths." Philadelphia: University of Pennsylvania, 2005. actionforhappiness.org/media/52486/340_ways_to_use_character_ strengths.pdf.

References

Rethorst, Chad D., Bradley M. Wipfli, and Daniel M. Landers. "The Antidepressive Effects of Exercise." *Sports Medicine* 39, no. 6 (2009): 491–511.

Rogge, Timothy. "Panic Disorder." Medline Plus, March 10, 2014. nlm.nih .gov/medlineplus/ency/article/000924.htm.

Shafran, Roz, Zafra Cooper, and Christopher G. Fairburn. "Clinical Perfectionism: A Cognitive-Behavioural Analysis." *Behaviour Research and Therapy* 40, no. 7 (2002): 773–91.

Smith, Ronald E., and Irwin G. Sarason. "Social Anxiety and the Evaluation of Negative Interpersonal Feedback." *Journal of Consulting and Clinical Psychology* 43, no. 3 (1975): 429.

Tafarodi, Romin W., and William B. Swann Jr. "Self-Liking and Self-Competence as Dimensions of Global Self-Esteem: Initial Validation of a Measure." *Journal of Personality Assessment* 65, no. 2 (1995): 322–42.

Tolin, David F. "Is Cognitive-Behavioral Therapy More Effective Than Other Therapies?: A Meta-Analytic Review." *Clinical Psychology Review* 30, no. 6 (2010): 710–20.

Vohs, Kathleen D., Roy F. Baumeister, Brandon J. Schmeichel, Jean M. Twenge, Noelle M. Nelson, and Dianne M. Tice. "Making Choices Impairs Subsequent Self-Control: A Limited-Resource Account of Decision Making, Self-Regulation, and Active Initiative." *Journal of Personality and Social Psychology* 94, no. 5 (2008): 883.

Wells, Adrian. *Metacognitive Therapy for Anxiety and Depression*. New York: Guilford Press, 2011.

Winch, Guy. *Emotional First Aid: Practical Strategies for Treating Failure, Rejection, Guilt, and Other Everyday Psychological Injuries*. New York: Exisle, 2013.

Young, Jeffrey, and Janet Klosko. *Reinventing Your Life: The Breakthrough Program to End Negative Behavior and Feel Great Again*. New York: Plume, 1994.

Young, Jeffrey, Janet Klosko, and Marjorie Weishaar. *Schema Therapy: A Practitioner's Guide*. New York: Guilford Press, 2003.

NOTES

Chapter 1

1 "Facts & Statistics."

2 Butler et al., "The Empirical Status of Cognitive-Behavioral Therapy"; Hofmann and Smits, "Cognitive-Behavioral Therapy for Adult Anxiety Disorders"; Tolin, "Is Cognitive-Behavioral Therapy More Effective Than Other Therapies?"

3 Norem and Chang, "The Positive Psychology of Negative Thinking."

Chapter 2

1 Kotov et al., "Linking 'Big' Personality Traits to Anxiety."

2 Aron and Aron, "Sensory-Processing Sensitivity."

3 Aron, *The Highly Sensitive Person*.

4 Halvorson and Higgins, *Focus*.

5 "Big Five Personality Traits."

6 Markman, "The Upside and Downside of Being Nice at Work."

7 Fry and Debats, "Perfectionism and the Five-Factor Personality Traits."

Chapter 3

1 Harvey, "A Cognitive Model of Insomnia."

2 Winch, *Emotional First Aid*.

3 McGonigal, "How to Make Stress Your Friend."

4 Tafarodi and Swann, "Self-Liking and Self-Competence as Dimensions of Global Self-Esteem."

Chapter 4

1 Dugas, Gosselin, and Ladouceur, "Intolerance of Uncertainty and Worry."

2 Markman, "Changing Habits Beautifully."

3 Dweck, *Mindset*.

4 Gollwitzer and Brandstätter, "Implementation Intentions and Effective Goal Pursuit."

5 "Intermittent Reinforcement."

6 Kramer, Guillory, and Hancock, "Experimental Evidence of Massive-Scale Emotional Contagion through Social Networks."

Chapter 5

1 "Need for Cognition."

2 Edwards, Rapee, and Franklin, "Postevent Rumination and Recall Bias for a Social Performance Event in High and Low Socially Anxious Individuals."

3 Wells, *Metacognitive Therapy for Anxiety and Depression*.

4 Lyubomirsky et al., "Ruminative Response Styles and Delay of Seeking Diagnosis for Breast Cancer Symptoms."

5 McGonigal, "Does Self-Compassion or Criticism Motivate Self-Improvement?"

6 Breines and Chen, "Self-Compassion Increases Self-Improvement Motivation."

7 McKay, Fanning, and Ona, *Mind and Emotions*.

8 Beck, *Cognitive Behavior Therapy*.

9 Hofmann et al., "The Effect of Mindfulness-Based Therapy on Anxiety and Depression."

10 Boyes, "5 Meditation Tips for Beginners."

11 Iyengar and Lepper, "When Choice Is Demotivating."

Chapter 6

1 Egan, Wade, and Shafran, "Perfectionism as a Transdiagnostic Process."

2 Young, Klosko, and Weishaar, *Schema Therapy.*

3 Shafran, Cooper, and Fairburn, "Clinical Perfectionism."

4 Elliott and Dweck, "Goals."

5 Mayer, McCormick, and Strong, "Mood-Congruent Memory and Natural Mood."

6 Markman, *Smart Thinking.*

7 Bernhard, "4 Tips for Slowing Down to Reduce Stress."

8 Vohs et al., "Making Choices Impairs Subsequent Self-Control."

Chapter 7

1 Rapee and Lim, "Discrepancy between Self- and Observer Ratings of Performance in Social Phobics."

2 Boyes and Fletcher, "Metaperceptions of Bias in Intimate Relationships."

3 Derrick, "Energized by Television."

4 Smith and Sarason, "Social Anxiety and the Evaluation of Negative Interpersonal Feedback."

5 Barrett et al., "Family Enhancement of Cognitive Style in Anxious and Aggressive Children."

6 Linehan, *Skills Training Manual for Treating Borderline Personality Disorder.*

Chapter 8

1 Aldao, Nolen-Hoeksema, and Schweizer, "Emotion-Regulation Strategies across Psychopathology."

2 Holahan et al., "Stress Generation, Avoidance Coping, and Depressive Symptoms."

3 Gottman and Silver, *The Seven Principles for Making Marriage Work.*

4 Leith and Baumeister, "Empathy, Shame, Guilt, and Narratives of Interpersonal Conflicts"; Baumeister, Stillwell, and Heatherton, "Guilt."

5 Brown, "Listening to Shame."

6 Glenn et al., "Who Gets the Most out of Cognitive Behavioral Therapy for Anxiety Disorders?"

7 Feske and Chambless, "Cognitive Behavioral Versus Exposure Only Treatment for Social Phobia."

8 Allen, *Getting Things Done*.

9 See "Undo Sending Your Mail," support.google.com/mail/answer/1284885?hl=en.

10 Boyes, "7 Ways You Can Benefit from Procrastinating."

Chapter 9

1 Rethorst, Wipfli, and Landers, "The Antidepressive Effects of Exercise."

2 Holt-Lunstad, Birmingham, and Light, "Influence of a 'Warm Touch.'"

Chapter 10

1 See "Test How Self-Compassionate You Are," self-compassion.org/test-your-self-compassion-level.html.

2 Rogge, "Panic Disorder."

3 Linehan, Bohus, and Lynch, "Dialectical Behavior Therapy for Pervasive Emotion Dysregulation."

4 Linehan, *Skills Training Manual for Treating Borderline Personality Disorder*.

5 Masuda et al., "Cognitive Defusion and Self-Relevant Negative Thoughts."

6 Arch et al., "Randomized Clinical Trial of Cognitive Behavioral Therapy (CBT) Versus Acceptance and Commitment Therapy (ACT) for Mixed Anxiety Disorders."

7 Gould, Ott, and Pollack, "A Meta-Analysis of Treatment Outcome for Panic Disorder."

8 "Coping with Physical Alarms"; "Panic Stations."

Chapter 11

1 Rashid and Anjum, "340 Ways to Use VIA Character Strengths."

2 Young and Klosko, *Reinventing Your Life.*

3 Padesky, "Schema Change Processes in Cognitive Therapy."

4 Murray, Holmes, and Griffin, "The Self-Fulfilling Nature of Positive Illusions in Romantic Relationships."

INDEX

Page numbers in **bold** indicate tables; those in *italics* indicate flowcharts.

Index

Index

Index

Index

Index